D1368787

A Physician Faces Cancer in Himself

A Physician Faces Cancer
in Himself

SAMUEL SANES, M.D.

State University of New York Press

ALBANY

This book was first published as a series of
articles in THE BUFFALO PHYSICIAN beginning
with the issue of Summer 1974 and ending
with Fall 1978.

First published in book form in 1979 by
State University of New York Press
Albany, New York

Printed in the United States of America

Library of Congress Cataloging in Publication Data

Sanes, Samuel.
    A physician faces cancer in himself.

    Originally published in the Buffalo physician, Summer 1974-Fall
1978.
    1. Reticulum cell sarcoma—Biography. 2. Physicians—New York
(State)—Buffalo—Biography. I. Title. II. Title: Disseminated reticulum cell sarcoma. [DNLM: 1. Sarcoma, Reticulum cell—Personal
narratives. WH525 S223p]
RC280.L9S36   362.1'9'699409   [B]   79-13124
ISBN 0-87395-395-9

Contents

Foreword

To Dr. Samuel Sanes, all of life was a learning experience.

And because he was, first and foremost, a teacher, what he learned he wanted to share.

Hence this book, which originated with a series of articles written for *The Buffalo Physician,* quarterly alumni publication of the School of Medicine of the State University of New York at Buffalo.

Dr. Sanes' accomplishments over the years were many, but teaching always came first.

During more than 30 years on the faculty of the School of Medicine, he taught pathology to most of the physicians and dentists practicing in Buffalo today, as well as many of the nurses and medical technologists.

He received both of the school's official awards for teaching, the Dean's and the Stockton Kimball Awards.

More significantly, he was repeatedly honored by the classes he taught.

One, in dedicating its yearbook to him, cited his "dynamic teaching of the subject matter of pathology," but stressed that his greatest contribution was his "philosophy of medicine and life in general."

Another presented him with a framed hand-lettered and illuminated copy of what the Lebanese poet, Kahlil Gibran, said about teaching in "The Prophet":

"No man can reveal to you aught but that which already lies half asleep in the dawning of your knowledge.

"The teacher who walks in the shadow of the temple, among his followers, gives not of his wisdom but rather of his faith and his lovingness.

"If he is indeed wise he does not bid you enter the house of his wisdom, but rather leads you to the threshold of your own mind."

An alumnus of an earlier class, chief of surgery in a large hospital and a teacher himself, recalled what it had been like to be one of Dr. Sanes' students in a letter written after he learned of his illness:

"Your surgical and autopsy pathology conferences were like a spot of sunshine in a stormy week. Your humorous and live way of bringing out a point and keeping our attention interested me in teaching and influenced my style, even now.

"You knew and recognized us as individuals, even by name frequently. . . . The memory of your warm, loving and lovable relationships with your students continues to inspire me."

Dr. Sanes never lost interest in the men and women who had been his students. He took pride in their accomplishments, sympathized with them in their times of difficulty.

Many continued to come to him with their problems, as they had when they were in medical school.

In the often discouraging days of his illness, letters, phone calls and visits from former students were bright punctuation marks.

He had always felt that education of the public was as much a part of his responsibility as a physician as education of members of the health profession.

For many years he averaged one or more lectures a week on subjects as diverse as cancer control, medicine in art and music, the medical investigation of crime.

He was a long-time moderator of the University's Medical Round Table on WBEN and WBEN-TV and co-ordinator of the station's pioneering television program, Modern Medicine, in 1953-56.

For none of these contributions did he ever ask or accept a fee.

But he was more than a teacher. Like Benjamin Franklin, whom he much admired, he was a universal man.

"Medicine is part of the entire fabric of life and nothing can be foreign or alien to a physician," he said once.

A founder of the Erie County Unit of the American Cancer Society, he served twice as its president and as president of the society's State Division.

He was president of the Erie County Medical Society, the New York State Society of Pathologists, the New York State Association of Public Health Laboratories.

For eight years he served as a member of the Medical Grievance Committee of the New York State Board of

Regents and for two as a member of the New York State Board of Medicine.

He was president of the Jewish Center of Buffalo and the New York State Section of the National Jewish Welfare Board.

There was still time for private enjoyment—travel, reading, modern art, music from Beethoven to John Cage, jazz, even rock. His mind was never closed to the new and different.

In 1953 The *Buffalo Evening News* named him one of his city's "outstanding citizens."

He had been retired less than two years and married only 15 months when he learned, in February, 1973, that he had an incurable type of cancer—reticulum cell sarcoma or histiocytic lymphoma.

Theretofore he had seen cancer from the viewpoint of a student, a pathologist, a Cancer Society volunteer. Now, seeing it as a patient, he realized how much he still had to learn.

On his visits to the lymphoma-leukemia clinic at Roswell Park Memorial Institute he made notes—of his own experiences and those related to him by fellow patients and their families.

The editor of *The Buffalo Physician*, learning of this, suggested that he write an article about it. He wrote one, discovered that he still had more to say, and ended up writing a series. It brought widespread response from former students all over the country.

He never missed a deadline though, as his disease progressed, writing became increasingly difficult.

At the time of his diagnosis, he had been told that 76% of patients with his disease died within two years.

He lived five years and five months.

Until the last year, all of his treatment was as an ambulatory outpatient. He was never hospitalized except overnight, for diagnostic tests.

In the beginning his major complaints were due to the side effects of treatment—radiation therapy, chemotherapy and experimental immunotherapy.

He suffered perversion of taste, nausea, loss of hair and overwhelming exhaustion.

The exhaustion persisted, coupled with muscular pain and weakness, after his disease was in remission.

In late 1976 and early 1977 his blood picture deteriorated steadily.

His hematocrit, normally more than 40, had dropped to 35 after radiation. Now it fell to 25. His white blood count fell to 2800—normal values are 4000-10,000; his platelet count to 45,000 as compared with a normal of 150,000-400,000.

In August, 1977, he entered the institute for a splenectomy which his physicians hoped would improve things.

It didn't, except briefly.

Soon he was receiving biweekly transfusions of red blood cells for his anemia. His blood platelets were agglutinated and there was constant danger that a blood vessel might be obstructed by the clumped cells. His white cell count climbed to 42,000.

He had daily fever, often accompanied by shaking chills, and dypsnea on exertion. The generalized muscular pain and weakness persisted.

In 1978 he was hospitalized four times, for periods ranging from one to four weeks.

By now he was so weak that he required assistance to get out of bed, even to turn from side to side. He couldn't get in or out of the bath tub, dress in street clothes, walk upstairs without support.

When he slipped and fell to the living room floor his wife had to telephone the rescue squad to get help in lifting him up.

His sight deteriorated. He developed persistent hiccups. During one hospitalization an apparent small stroke left him aphasic for several hours. Although there were no residual neurologic defects, the fear of losing permanently his ability to communicate haunted him.

Through it all he continued to write. When he could no longer do so in longhand because of his muscular weakness, he dictated his initial draft to his wife while lying in bed. She typed it, returned it to him for editing, then retyped it with his suggested changes.

He entered the hospital for the last time June 22. In the following days his temperature occasionally spiked as high as 105. The hiccups persisted. He was restless and unable to sleep, even with sedation.

On June 26, his 72nd birthday, he read the proofs of his final article for *The Buffalo Physician*. Still hopeful that somehow the relentless advance of his disease might be slowed down he arranged to illustrate it with pictures of himself undergoing physical therapy.

Two weeks later—long before the journal was published—he was dead.

Autopsy indicated that his original disease was still largely in remission. There were only two small foci of malignant lymphoma in the left lower lung lobe and the mesentery.

In the last months, however, he had developed another malignancy—chronic myelocytic leukemia.

The immediate cause of death was cardiorespiratory failure and sepsis from multiple abscesses in the left lung, micro-abscesses in the liver, pyelonephritis involving both kidneys.

A fellow physician wrote his wife:

"None of us can share your sorrow but all of us share your loss."

Mildred Spencer Sanes

A Physician Faces Cancer in Himself

1

Discovery and Early Reactions

The pathologist didn't hedge as he had in the hospital the day before, after examining the frozen sections.

"I've seen your paraffin sections," he told me. "You have a malignant lymphoma, of the mixed cell or reticulum cell sarcoma type."

"That's it . . . that's the end," I thought. And then, aloud, "Maybe I'll not make my next birthday."

The pathologist, a former student of mine and a colleague and friend of 31 years, had volunteered to be the one among my physicians to tell me. He had come to my home after work.

Perhaps he thought it would be easier for me to hear the news from him.

He made a couple of attempts to console me, but didn't raise any false hopes. His eyes seemed to say compassionately, "Poor son-of-a-bitch."

He stayed a few minutes, then excused himself. His wife, he told me, was waiting dinner. They had guests.

My wife had gone out briefly on an errand. Since yesterday she had been clinging wishfully to the pathologist's impression from the frozen sections that "non-specific inflammatory hyperplasia" was a possible diagnosis.

She would be coming home soon. I would have to tell her the final verdict.

I had found the first small lump, about the size of a lima bean, while bathing. It was on the left side of my chest, posterior to the left axilla.

Nervously I palpated the rest of my body.

I found a smaller lump in the mid-pubic region, and another in the postero-lateral aspect of the upper part of the right arm.

All were superficial, discrete, moveable. The lumps on the left side of the chest and in the mid-pubic region were firm; that in the right upper arm resilient. The only palpable lymph nodes were located in both inguinal regions. They were small, the right slightly larger than the left.

Physicians whom I consulted minimized the possibility of malignant tumor. Along with the physical findings, the sites were unlikely ones.

At my insistence, however, they agreed to biopsy the lesion on the left side of my chest. There was no point, they maintained, in biopsying the other lumps.

After the biopsy and the diagnosis of reticulum cell sarcoma I had a complete diagnostic workup—from urinalysis and blood count to lymphangiograms and a total body gallium scan. The scan showed involvement of mediastinal lymph nodes. Ten months later, after needle aspiration proved suggestive, a second biopsy, of the mid-pubic lump, which had not increased in size, confirmed reticulum cell sarcoma there too. Needle aspirations of the right inguinal nodes were negative.

I had retired at 65 from the practice and teaching of pathology.

Since I was entering a new phase of my life, I thought it advisable to have a thorough physical checkup.

Until then I had been in what I judged acceptable health. Although I felt some fatigue at the end of the day's work, I told myself that this was normal with increasing age. My internist had diagnosed a pain in my left shoulder and arm, which was not incapacitating, as due to arthritis of the cervical spine.

The physical examination that I underwent in the fall of 1971 was a thorough one, from scalp to soles. It included X-ray studies of my chest, GI and GU tracts, bones and joints, an electrocardiogram, laboratory tests focused on my blood, heart, arteries, kidneys and liver.

The examining physician gave me a clean bill of health except for the previously detected cervical arthritis, for which he prescribed no specific treatment. He advised me to go ahead with the plans I had made for retirement. I could do anything, he said.

Now, 17 months later, in February, 1973, I had a definitive diagnosis of disseminated reticulum cell sarcoma.

Someone has said that cancer is a lonely disease. It is especially so if the victim is a physician, above all if he is a pathologist whose outlook is influenced by the destructive and fatal results of the disease as he has seen them at autopsy.

No one who hasn't faced cancer in himself can truly imagine what a cancer patient is experiencing. Even those closest to the patient, who love him, can only sympathize. They can't empathize.

The patient feels that empathy with other cancer patients, particularly those with the same type and stage of cancer as his. But even with them he is alone. In the last analysis, the question of his own well-being and survival is instinctively of primary concern.

Individual reactions toward disease and death spring from individual minds and hearts. They depend on various factors in one's personal life situation, character and personality, social and cultural background, what one knows about his disease.

How one meets a diagnosis of cancer is also related to his age at the time the disease is diagnosed, occupation, family, financial status, philosophical and religious beliefs.

The type and extent of the cancer, the attitudes of the attending physicians, the kind and efficacy of treatment, are of fundamental importance.

Take patients with three different types of cancer:

—Squamous cell carcinoma-in-situ of the cervix.

—Mature adenocarcinoma of the recto-sigmoid, showing superficial invasion of the bowel wall and microscopic metastases to regional nodes.

—Disseminated reticulum cell sarcoma.

Each will have an altogether different outlook to his

disease if he understands the pathologic and therapeutic significance of the diagnosis.

But even when the pathologic diagnosis, including distribution and histologic grade, and the treatment are the same, no two patients react in exactly the same way.

Suppose a 65-year-old steel worker and a 29-year-old dentist are both told that they have disseminated reticulum cell sarcoma.

The steel worker's wife is dead, his children grown and married. He can retire and live comfortably on his pension and social security. He has adequate health insurance. He has a firm faith in his religion and its promise of an after-life.

According to vital statistics, he knows that his life expectancy is running out anyway.

"I'll be happy to settle for five years," he confesses.

The dentist has just started in practice after a residency in orthodontics. He is in debt. His life and disability insurance portfolio has not been completed. He does have Social Security credit.

He and his wife are the parents of three children under six years of age.

He remembers just enough from his sophomore course in general pathology to view his disease in its darkest aspects. He is skeptical about all religion and has no faith at all in a life after death.

Before his diagnosis, the life expectancy tables had told him that the average healthy man of his age had 40 to 45 years to live.

Despite the disease that they have in common, each patient will face his reticulum cell sarcoma, and the

5

future, alone—on the basis of his individual human situation.

The cancer patient has not only a medical problem but a semantic one.

Medically cancer means a particular lesion in a particular person at a particular time and place.

Semantically, however, the word "cancer" signifies more than it denotes medically.

It carries terrifying connotations accumulated over the centuries when it was practically 100% untreatable, incurable, fatal.

"We should discard the term 'cancer,'" an old general practitioner once told me. "We could make progress in clinical management and save time and money in public education if we called the disease a name free of the old connotations, reflective of current accomplishments and future hopes."

He pointed out the value, in his own time, of the replacements in medical and public usage of the term "consumption" by "tuberculosis."

Test yourself by playing a word-association game. Is your spontaneous response to "Wilms' tumor" as negative as that to "cancer of the kidney?"

Yet the actual lesion referred to, regardless of its name, is a curable one today.

The first three months after my diagnosis of reticulum cell sarcoma were the hardest for me, as some other patients say they were for them. They were devoted

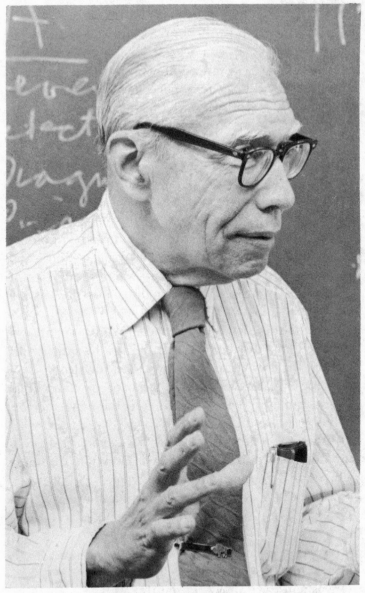

Dr. Sanes lectures to a sophomore pathology class on what he has learned as a patient.

largely to treatment, follow-up examinations and resting at home.

I chose treatment and followup in Roswell Park Memorial Institute, a national center for lymphoma-leukemia. My internist received regular reports from the institute.

After my diagnostic workup, my physicians prescribed 4½ weeks of daily supervoltage mantle radiation. They also put me on an experimental program of immunotherapy with periodic intradermal BCG vaccination.

In late November, after a positive biopsy report on the second lump in the mid-pubic region, chemotherapy was prescribed. Following two intravenous injections of vincristine, I went on a daily maintenance dose of 150 milligrams of Cytoxan.

Before treatment, I had no complaints apparently referable to my disease except the lumps. I was active all day, met the normal social obligations, traveled.

Except for inflammation at the site of injection, I had no noticeable untoward reactions to the BCG vaccine. Radiation was a different story.

During those first three months, my physical problems all seemed traceable to the radiation treatment rather than any underlying disease.

I lost the hair in the posterior portion of my scalp and my beard in the submaxillary and anterior cervical areas.

I experienced loss and perversion of my sense of taste, and my appetite diminished.

I was nauseated fairly constantly.

My mouth was dry and pharyngitis made it painful to swallow.

The skin in my axillae moistened and desquamated.

I lost 15 pounds of weight.

My hematocrit, white blood cell and platelet counts, which were checked three times a week, dropped.

I experienced fatigue that limited my performance of daily activities.

In June I developed shingles, with fever of 101-102. Later in the summer I suffered symptoms in my left shoulder, arm and hand which were interpreted as a possible variant of Lhermite syndrome.

From my own experience, and from observing fellow patients, I have learned much about the problems that confront the patient with disseminated lymphoma. (Problems, of course, vary in number, kind and degree with different patients.)

The disease and its treatment will be a monkey on the patient's back for the rest of his life.

It is potentially fatal. Survival is a matter of general percentages. No one can give a 100% guarantee of cure. The patient may live months, or many years. He now observes two birthdays—the most important being the anniversary of his diagnosis, marking the years of survival.

The disease is chronic. There are all sorts of possible manifestations and complications.

To the healthy person, even if he is no longer young, the future seems infinite. With a diagnosis of disseminated lymphoma, a curtain drops across it. Life becomes a matter of day-to-day planning. Goals are short-term ones, scaled down, limited. Looking back is more tempting than looking forward.

Treatment, whether radiation, chemotherapy or immunotherapy, can have side effects that are more disfiguring, discomforting and dangerous than the disease itself. Measures adopted to prevent and counteract these side effects may cause side effects of their own.

Follow-up visits to his physicians, the hospital or cancer institute may be scheduled daily, then weekly or biweekly. A longer span becomes a welcome reprieve.

There is gratitude for a remission and despair over a relapse or resistance to further therapy.

Personal and interpersonal strains and stresses are numerous.

The ambulatory patient may be dependent on others, usually relatives, for transportation to and from the place of treatment. The homebound patient may be dependent upon his family for more intimate types of care.

If the patient is unable to keep a steady job, because of the disease itself, the effects of treatment or the schedule of treatment and checkups, he may feel that he no longer has a purpose in life.

To the university student, in whom lymphoma-leukemia is the most frequent cancer, the disease can mean the interruption, or the end, of his studies and his career.

Many patients have to curtail social, recreational, organizational and community activities.

Retirement or change to a less demanding job will

mean financial problems for many patients. Medical and hospital care doesn't come cheap to the person or family who must pay all or a major portion of the charges. And the costs can rise even higher if a patient has to go out of town for treatment and pay for transportation and room and board in a hotel, motel or rooming house.

The person with disseminated lymphoma takes on a new occupation, that of patient. He can never retire from it and cannot escape, even when on vacation.

Before taking a trip he may have to arrange to see a physician or physicians at intervals during his absence from home.

His itinerary or vacation spot will be determined by the availability and accessibility of medical and laboratory facilities.

He will need regular physical checkups, blood counts, X-ray films. Perhaps, depending on the results, his treatment will have to be modified.

The patient who is on drug therapy takes his drugs with him. His carry-on flight bag is a portable pharmacy. With his passport and tourist visa he carries a letter from his physician describing his disease and bearing diagnostic and therapeutic instructions for the physicians who will look after him while he is away from home.

He may have to produce that letter for customs officials who ask "Are you carrying any drugs?"

Along with physical death, the patient with disseminated reticulum cell sarcoma faces social death, death as an active, contributing, accepted member of society. The latter may seem much the worse fate to him.

In the first three months after my diagnosis, while my physicians and I sought to ward off physical death by treatment, I also fought the mental and emotional battle against social death.

My weapons were what I came to think of as the "three A's"—acceptance of my disease, adjustment to it, and assurance—the latter dependent on the attention, notice, understanding, and sympathy of others.

Most patients accept the diagnosis of malignant lymphoma by biopsy without question.

A rare patient may never accept it, denying his disease to the point of disregarding the prognosis and refusing treatment.

A certain number of patients delay acceptance of the diagnosis until they get an additional opinion on the microscopic changes.

They are aware of the kind of treatment and prognosis involved in a diagnosis of malignant lymphoma and of the possibility of diagnostic error. (Witness the various lesions classified as "pseudo lymphomas.")

It is not easy even for a pathologist who trusts the professional expertise of his colleagues to accept such a diagnosis.

In my own case, I asked the pathologist who first read the slides to have other pathologists look at them. I was sure that as a friend and colleague of many years he would feel better about sharing the responsibility.

Even when the other pathologists concurred fully in

his findings, I didn't feel altogether comfortable until I had microscopically examined the slides myself.

Successful adjustment to the fact that one has disseminated lymphoma doesn't come automatically with the acceptance of the diagnosis and its implications.

A fellow patient in his 20s demonstrated this vividly during two successive visits to the lymphoma-leukemia clinic.

On his first visit he was obviously anxious and agitated.

Sitting next to him was a calm, poised, healthy-looking girl, also in her 20s. She told him that she was waiting for a follow-up examination for lymphoma, diagnosed four years earlier.

"Four years—that's good!" the young fellow exclaimed. "The doctor told me just last week that I have cancer of the lymph nodes. I can hardly believe it. I'm awfully scared."

A week later the same patient was asked by the clinic physician who had seen him originally, and explained cancer of the lymph nodes (Hodgkin's Disease) to him:

"How are you today?"

"Well," the patient responded, "I'm now accepting the fact that I have cancer. But I'm still awfully scared."

The physical battle against disseminated lymphoma consists of following the prescribed regimen, with whatever discomforts or limitations it implies.

It is a simple and straightforward conflict.

Not so the mental and emotional struggle.

Some patients with disseminated lymphoma may adjust to their disease, mentally and emotionally, as other patients do to duodenal ulcer or diverticulosis of the colon.

They must be few.

For the average patient, lymphoma is the most serious crisis he has ever had to go through.

He must combat a host of fearful thoughts and feelings. These include uncertainty, inadequacy, isolation, recognition of his mortality, guilt, anxiety, depression, withdrawal, even, for some, the temptation of suicide.

Each must find for himself the weapons that are most effective.

How rapidly and successfully he routs the enemy depends on the factors I have previously mentioned—the strengths and weaknesses of his own personality, his philosophical and religious attitudes toward life and death, and the support he receives from family, friends, professional colleagues and co-workers, fellow cancer patients.

If he still needs help, there are trained professionals to whom he can turn—his own physicians, nurses, social workers, clergymen and, if need be, psychiatrists.

It is not an easy battle. But victory on the mental and emotional front, when and if achieved, can be even more satisfying than winning the physical fight.

Life has a way of setting a man back on his heels.

Throughout my adult life I had imagined how I

would face and cope with a final illness, such as cancer, when it came.

For more than 25 years I had been a public education speaker for my county and state cancer societies. During those years I had talked to thousands of healthy men, women and children about how to meet cancer in themselves or their families.

For ten years, as chairman of a hospital tumor clinic, I had counseled patients with all types and stages of cancer.

Yet now that I had to cope with the reality of disseminated reticulum cell sarcoma in myself I was like the actor who is seized with stage fright on opening night.

After weeks of rehearsals, his role letter and gesture perfect, he is seemingly prepared for any contingency. Then, in the face of a critical first night audience, he panics.

The actor conquers his fears in a few seconds and goes on serenely, in reflex to his preparation.

That was not true for me.

In past mental and emotional crises, less serious to be true, I had relied on reason for my weapon and had not been disappointed.

In this new crisis, reason failed to allay and dispel my fearful thoughts and feelings with the speed with which an antibiotic inhibits and destroys pathogenic bacteria.

I became increasingly self-preoccupied.

My fears were not so much for my life but for the loss of all that had made life worthwhile and enjoyable— useful work, multiple interests, professional and personal relations.

"Why can't I adjust?" I asked myself over and over again.

"Why doesn't reason conquer this problem as quickly and effectively as it has conquered others for me? Why do the worries that I think I have put aside during the daytime, the fears that I think I have overcome, still keep me awake at night or stalk me in my dreams?"

A fellow patient in her 50s who also has disseminated reticulum cell sarcoma provided me with the insight I should have possessed as a physician.

"It's not easy," she consoled me. "I always prided myself on being able to accept things and adjust to them. But no amount of reasoning seemed to help me when I first had to adjust to the reality that I had cancer. I was shattered. I went through a nightmare. It takes reason and determination—but it also takes time."

My battle, like hers, was won with time.

Time, I found, is not only a medium in which reason can neutralize the potency of fears. It also, in itself, acts as a diluent.

As I approached the end of the first three months after my diagnosis, my thinking and feeling became more positive.

I sought for optimism justified by available scientific data and experience—and for hope founded on a reasonable projection of that data and experience into the future.

On that basis I made realistic deductions regarding possible remission and survival.

I didn't look for headline breakthroughs or miracles, but I left an opening for the unexpected. I recalled that the application of nitrogen mustard against lymphoma came from an accidental discovery during World War II.

Without becoming a Pollyanna, I ceased being a Gloomy Gus.

I determined to continue living and enduring, to make the best of life within the limits imposed by my disease, to fulfill, as far as I could, my personal and social roles.

Retirement, I learned, had many advantages for me in coping with my disease mentally and emotionally. I had already changed my way of life from a rigidly scheduled work orientation to a more relaxed program. I could continue that at my own time and pace.

The patient with disseminated lymphoma can never forget his disease, but he need not let it take over all aspects of his life.

As he adjusts to life with its limitations—through reason and determination or, as many do, through faith and prayer—he also adjusts to death.

No matter how self-sufficient he may have been before his disease was diagnosed, the patient with disseminated lymphoma can't win the battle alone.

He needs to feel that despite the fact that he has cancer—and the changes cancer makes in his life—he is still part of the world of the living, recognized, appreciated and loved.

In ordinary social contacts I have never been considered a "hale fellow well-met."

Some persons, I am sure, have looked on me as a loner, despite my full life in professional, organizational and community activities.

17

During previous benign, self-limited illnesses I remained self-sufficient enough to think that "He suffers best who suffers alone."

But in adjusting to disseminated reticulum cell sarcoma, particularly during those first three months, I found that the opposite is true.

"When you go through the desert, it is much better to have someone with you."

Like most cancer sufferers, I needed the assurance of others. I wanted desperately to be remembered by family, friends, professional colleagues and co-workers.

A fellow cancer patient in her 60s expressed it for me.

She had arrived at the cancer institute after a 200-mile automobile trip, gone through the admissions procedure and was waiting in her wheelchair to be taken to the ward.

Pale, weary from the journey, her abdomen distended from her disease, she reached out to touch the arm of one of her family who had accompanied her and was now leaving for home.

"Please," she begged, "don't forget me."

2

Responses of Lay Persons and Physicians to Patients with Cancer

"Please don't forget me!"

Many times during the three months after my diagnosis of disseminated reticulum cell sarcoma and the onset of radiation therapy the words of that other cancer patient echoed in my memory.

She had sensed what I was to learn as the weeks passed.

Forgetting the chronically ill—especially those with disseminated cancer—is easy for those who are chronically healthy.

For most adult Americans, health is a matter of first priority.

"As long as you've got your health," we say, "that's the most important thing."

Indeed few of us want to think of disease, let alone face it in ourselves or in others.

When we do respond to disease in another person, we do so best when his illness is one that leads to recovery or cure after five to ten days in the hospital and a brief convalescence at home—when we know that he will be returning to a full schedule of work, family responsibilities, social and community activities.

A medical example of such an illness would be pneumococcus pneumonia treated with penicillin; a surgical one, cholecystitis and cholelithiasis treated by cholecystectomy.

Let us follow a 60-year-old man as he goes through an uneventful post-operative course after cholecystectomy.

He gets a surfeit of attention from everyone.

Into his hospital room flows a constant stream of greeting cards, flowers, candy, fruit, wine, telephone calls and visitors.

The traffic in and out of his room may become so heavy that the physician, to protect him from getting overtired, will order a "no visitors" sign hung on the door.

Even this won't discourage some of the well-wishers. They'll ignore the sign and sneak in to cheer the patient with the buoyant expression of their best wishes.

This continues throughout the ten days of his stay.

He will probably be up and moving around the room on the second or third day after the operation.

He puts aside the coarse white hospital gown and dons the colorful new pajamas and robe his wife has gone out and purchased for his trip to the hospital.

Sitting up in bed, or in a chair, he receives the

tributes of relatives, friends, professional colleagues, and co-workers like a king from his subjects.

It's all very assuring, very satisfying to the ego.

When the time comes to go home, the patient may even feel a little regretful that his time in the limelight has come to an end.

At home his boss or the personnel manager of the company where he is employed may visit or telephone him.

"Don't hurry back to work," they'll say. "Stay home until you are entirely well. Take a brief vacation if you need one. We'll wait for you." (They know that no matter what they say he'll be back on the job at the first possible moment.)

But what of the patient who has a cholecystectomy and doesn't go home in ten days, whose recovery isn't uneventful, whose post-operative course is complicated and who requires a protracted stay in the hospital?

Suppose this 60-year-old patient, shortly before his scheduled discharge from the hospital, develops a "stroke" due to cerebral thrombosis. He is left with facial paralysis and hemiplegia.

All too soon he and his wife find that the attention he enjoyed during his first seven to ten days in the hospital is degradable.

The flowers wilt, the candy and fruit are eaten, the wine drunk. The telephone rings less frequently.

The visitors stop coming. The occasional person who does drop in enters the room reluctantly and departs as quickly as possible. He has little to say.

There are fewer and fewer greeting cards. (Have you

ever tried to buy a card for a patient who isn't going to "have a speedy recovery" or "get well soon"?)

As time drags on, matters worsen. If the patient is transferred to an extended care facility or a nursing home, few but his immediate family will continue to keep in touch. And even some of them will begin to find excuses for not telephoning or visiting.

When the patient fails to come back to work in a short time, his employer will get restless, inform him that his sick leave has run out, that he is off the regular payroll, that he is released completely.

Although the patient is still in the world, he is not of it.

This is as true of a physician who becomes chronically ill as it is of a layman.

I watched it happen to an obstetrician-gynecologist who was a long-time friend.

A short time after he developed a mild Parkinson's syndrome, he was peremptorily forced out of a group practice by the two younger associates he had taken in when they completed training.

Of course, they were right that he should not have continued to deliver babies and operate.

But they might have acted with more consideration, keeping him on for tasks within his capabilities. The older man's mind was still keen and alert despite his neurologic impairment which itself was treatable.

Few Americans respond with understanding to chronic, lingering disease in other persons. This is particularly true if the disease is physically disfiguring and disabling, mind-altering, without specific therapy, irreversible, progressive, recurring, potentially fatal.

Diseases which meet these criteria include, besides "stroke," obstructive lung disease with diffuse emphysema and fibrosis, multiple sclerosis and disseminated cancer.

Patients with disseminated cancer carry the heaviest burden. Their disease has not only many of the "unattractive" characteristics mentioned above—it also has its name. The stigma of the word "cancer" and its connotations are from the very beginning more repelling to most persons than the actual characteristics of the disease itself.

My own cancer, disseminated reticulum cell sarcoma, has required no hospitalization except overnight stays for two biopsies and following a lymphangiogram. In the first three months, though, I was confined to my home much of the time.

During this period I was not dependent physically on others.

Psychologically, however, I did need assurance that I was still part of life.

I didn't want to feel forgotten, discarded, cut off from the real world.

Why, I wondered, did so few persons who knew about my condition, including professional colleagues and co-workers, offer expressions of assurance? Why didn't I receive them even from those persons from whom, because of close, long-time association, I might have expected them?

23

Lay persons give varied reasons for not getting in touch with a patient afflicted with disseminated cancer. Some of them are undoubtedly true. But there are other reasons that they don't give, that they won't admit even to themselves.

First, the reasons that they give, usually to the wife or other members of the family rather than to the patient himself:

"I've been so busy. I just kept putting it off." (The patient, after all, will be there next week, next month or next year—if he is fortunate enough to be still alive.)

"I didn't know how much he knew about his condition . . . what to say to him . . . whether he would want to talk about it." (My physicians at the cancer institute hadn't kidded me from the beginning about my condition. I would have been glad to discuss it openly. I found doing so helped me in adjusting to the disease.)

"It hurts me too much to see him. I've heard that his cancer is one of the bad ones. It must be awful living with that knowledge." (Gradually, although not easily, I adjusted to my prognosis in a realistic way.)

But what of the reasons people don't give, can't articulate?

A nurse with few illusions after long years of practice with cancer patients answered the question for me. Her own husband had had cancer, treated by surgery and radiation.

"People are cowards," she told me. "They're terrified merely by the word 'cancer.' They don't want to see sickness or suffering. They're upset just by the sight of a cancer patient, especially one with any visible effect of his disease or treatment—pallor, loss of weight, a mass in the neck. Some aren't sure that they may not catch the disease. They don't want to be reminded of death. Even thinking about it brings their own death closer. In regard to health and disease, life and death, they want to live in a closed world where everyone is healthy and sound, able and productive.''

Thus the patient with disseminated cancer, who must contend with his own fears, is deprived by the fears of the healthy of the assurance he so needs.

During the first three months after my diagnosis and the onset of radiation therapy I worried less about my disease and the side effects of treatment than I did about becoming isolated.

Somehow, I felt that if I could hold onto the outside world I would think and feel better. To me this meant especially the world of medicine. I didn't expect to participate in that world personally, for I had retired and I was ill, homebound, but I wanted to keep in touch with it through others, professional colleagues and co-workers. Conversation about things medical, if merely the latest gossip, seemed the most effective mood elevator, the best psychostimulant.

The mental-emotional lift from contact with one's professional world, whatever it may have been, holds even when a patient is bedridden, in pain, with terminal cancer.

TIME magazine reported the death from cancer of Charles E. Bohlen, former U.S. Ambassador to the

Soviet Union and retired State Department expert on Russian affairs. It told how Mr. Bohlen, in his last days of life, often in pain, responded with difficulty to most attempts at conversation. Yet a "visitor only needed to mention a scrap of news from Moscow or a question from Russian history and 'instantly as though by magic he would be his old, shrewd and endlessly knowledgeable self.'"

The physician-patient with disseminated cancer who wants to keep in touch with the world of medicine can do so best through other physicians.

But, unfortunately, physicians in general have the same hangups about cancer that lay persons do.

These hangups interfere with their relations to all disseminated cancer patients—relatives, friends, professional colleagues and co-workers not under their care as well as the patients for whose care they are responsible.

You might assume that physicians, because of their scientific training and background, would have a rational and objective view of cancer, the disease.

You might assume that as students in medical school and teaching hospitals they should have acquired a holistic and humane approach to their patients, one that would enable them to look on anyone with cancer as a sick person with a variety of problems and needs, thoughts and feelings.

But physicians are human beings too. They share all of the fears of lay persons. They're frightened by the very word "cancer." They envision themselves as potential victims. (My own reaction on first hearing my

diagnosis of reticulum cell sarcoma was one of hopelessness.)

But, in addition, disseminated cancer disturbs a physician of today for another reason. He knows that treatment of many such cancers, particularly in a progressive, recurring, terminal form, can offer no significant
remission or cure. Professionally the situation spells
defeat. Quite simply, in the context of his medical
education, training and philosophy, the physician cannot face this inevitable defeat.

There was a time, within my memory, when a physician had to accept defeat as normal and unavoidable.

When I was a junior medical student, I was taught
that the therapeutic function of the physician was a
three-fold one—to cure when possible, relieve when
indicated, comfort and console always.

The patient's recovery, if he was going to recover,
depended in many diseases on nature, not on his
physician. The important thing was not to interfere
with nature.

Limited in methods of diagnosis, too often with no
effective way of treating the diseases he could diagnose,
the physician concentrated on relieving complaints,
comforting and consoling the patient and his family.

In those days the "science of medicine" was embry-
onic. The "art of medicine" (the word "empathy" was
not yet in frequent usage) played a substantial part in
practice.

Today we have highly accurate techniques for detect-
ing disease and its complications in an early stage.

Treatment has become scientific instead of empiric. There are specific measures that can be taken to cure numerous diseases and complications. Complications can be prevented. Surgeons can even transplant vital organs. The physician doesn't have to depend on nature to do the job alone.

Because there is so much that he can do scientifically, the average physician now sees his therapeutic function differently than he did 50 years ago.

He looks at patients in terms of overcoming disease in as rapid a time as possible, or holding it in check over the long term.

He is liable to think less about relief and almost not at all about comfort and consolation.

With the waxing of the science of medicine, the art of medicine has waned.

Scientific medicine, however, may offer only meager help to many patients with disseminated cancer, likely none when the cancer is in a progressive, recurring, terminal form. The art of medicine can always be of aid.

But patients are deprived of its benefits because today's physicians have not learned it or deem it inappropriate to their self-image as scientific practitioners. They see their therapeutic function almost solely in terms of control, recovery, and cure. If treatment cannot achieve these goals, they feel defeated before they begin.

Their defeatist attitude may be communicated to the other members of the medical team who work with the patient—residents, interns, students, nurses, nurses' aides, even office secretaries.

They no longer think of the patient as a human being with thoughts, feelings, need for empathy and assurance. To them he is already as good as dead, and their manner reflects that feeling.

I don't want to be misunderstood. The role of the physician portrayed by Sir Luke Fildes in "The Doctor" is a thing of the past, and fortunately so, because of the tremendous advances in the science of medicine during the past 50-100 years.

Today no one would expect a busy physician to sit for hours, even days, at the bedside of a critically-ill patient for whom he could do little else.

However, it is not the quantity of time spent with such a patient that counts, but its quality.

Rapport, heedfulness, warmth, understanding can be communicated in a few words by a tone of voice, a smile, a touch.

The cancer patient may adapt to the fact that his physician cannot cure him or prolong his life. He cannot accept being disregarded emotionally. It crushes his spirit. And that applies to his family, too. (For palliation, empathy ought to rank with medical and surgical measures. An empathic physician can be the crucial factor in preventing a patient and his family from throwing away their time and money on quackery.)

Let us look at how certain physicians react to the persons who are their patients.

Take the surgeon who finds diffuse carcinoma of the pancreas with nodal, peritoneal and hepatic metastases when performing a laparotomy on a 55-year-old housewife.

He makes excuses for not stopping in after the operation to see the patient or talk to her anguished family. Making rounds with his resident, he leaves that patient until last. Then, after checking the chart at the nurses' station, he turns to the resident and remarks:

"There doesn't seem to be any change in this patient's condition. It's late. I have a full schedule at the office. Why don't you look in on her today? I'll see her on rounds tomorrow. . . ."

Often that tomorrow never comes. Rather than face the death he sees growing in the patient, the surgeon continues to find excuses to avoid her. He fails the woman and her family, who all need the assurance of his presence.

And then this advanced cancer patient goes home, perhaps with only a few months of life ahead of her. She becomes the responsibility of the internist who has been her personal physician for years and who referred her to the surgeon. As her disease worsens, her husband or some other member of the family calls the doctor.

The reply is terse:

"There's nothing further I can do. It's a waste of time for me to come to the house. I have responsibilities to my other patients . . . the ones I can help."

The circumstances in the foregoing case are not hypothetical.

The same sort of things can happen to a physician who has disseminated cancer.

I remember a physician in his 30s who developed what seemed to be an "acute abdomen." At operation it was found that he had widespread peritoneal metastases, apparently from an infiltrating carcinoma of the stomach.

The surgeon—on the faculty of a medical school and on the full-time staff of a teaching hospital where the patient had taken a residency—could not bear to discuss the patient's condition with him.

He avoided him in the hospital and failed to visit him on his return home.

The patient died in several months, embittered. He interpreted the surgeon's behavior not merely as a breach in personal relations but, in terms of medical ethics, as abandonment.

The development of medicine as a science, and the parallel growth of medical specialization, have affected the physician's awareness of each individual patient as a total human being. What is true for the patient with disseminated advanced cancer can also be true for the patient with a cancer that is diagnosed early, treated adequately and considered favorable for "cure."

A 44-year-old unmarried newspaper reporter in another city wrote to me, after undergoing a radical mastectomy for cancer of the breast with minimal axillary metastasis, "The surgeon says that I have 'healed beautifully.'"

Then she added wryly:

"Next week I'll be fitted for a prosthesis and will begin job hunting. In fact, I have a luncheon engagement this Friday with a prospective employer. My first public appearance since the operation. I'll have to wear a homemade stuffing, but maybe he won't notice.

"I suppose that when I start dating again, it will have to be with 90-year-old men.

"I'm just not getting as much done as I used to. Many nights I have just enough energy to flop into bed at 9:30. This isn't my idea of the way to live, and I'm going to do my best to change it. Next week I begin psychiatric counseling at a comprehensive care center, the name of which I've obtained through the local cancer society."

The surgeon who had operated upon the reporter had little or no awareness of his patient as a woman with all of the problems she faced. He didn't see the still-open mental and emotional wounds that she bore from her disease and treatment. It was enough that the surgical wound had "healed beautifully."

Medical education, in schools and hospitals, gives students a thorough exposure, orientation and training in regard to acute, controllable, recoverable and curable diseases, especially organic ones.

But how well does it prepare them, through regular assignment and follow-up of patients, through precept and example from clinical instructors, to care for human beings with chronic "incurable" diseases, for example, disseminated cancer?

Some time ago a physician and medical educator gave me one answer to this question.

At his school the head of the department of medicine

had proposed dividing the service in a large public teaching hospital into two parts.

One would consist of acute, active, "interesting" cases, "those you can do something for," and the other of chronic cases with little or no chance of improvement, "the crocks," who are "poor teaching material."

The former group would be assigned to the house staff and medical students. The latter would become in large measure the responsibility of part-time physicians hired from the community.

The proposal was never activated. Perhaps my informant exaggerated the whole thing to make a point.

But the view embodied in the proposal does exist, and, as a result, some, perhaps too many, medical school graduates look on time for chronic "incurable" patients as a useless or wasteful expenditure outside the therapeutic function of the modern physician.

Don't get me wrong. I realize that in what I've written about care and empathy for chronic "incurable" patients I may have done an injustice to today's medical education and practice by raising general implications on the basis of a few selected examples of individual medical educators, physicians and patients.

Please remember, however, that though not materially disabled or terminal, I'm a chronic "incurable" patient myself. For my disseminated cancer, the science of medicine offers no probable permanent cure and no predictable method of control. That's the personal standpoint from which I've been writing.

Further, with the exception of my immediate family, I

have felt closer to no one than to my fellow lymphoma patients who find themselves in the same leaky boat that I'm in. I've written also with them in mind. I have observed what empathic physicians, as well as other members of the medical team, mean to these men, women and children, whatever their general condition and prognosis. (Depending on his lesion, response to treatment, psychologic adjustment and luck, a patient with disseminated lymphoma can go for years in a relatively happy, useful life.)

May I submit in evidence again only a single, selected example, but one that I'm sure epitomizes the meaning of empathy to the chronic "incurable" patient.

A World War II veteran and college instructor with disseminated reticulum cell sarcoma sitting in the lymphoma-leukemia clinic comments:

"Isn't everyone nice here! They're cordial to you. They make you feel as if you're an individual, a person. They talk to you on your visits. They don't expect that you know everything. You go away feeling better—more than from pills. At the (name of out-of-town center deleted) they treat you like a guinea pig."

It's my impression (backed by a medical opinion poll of one State University of New York at Buffalo medical senior) that physicians trained in oncology who care for cancer patients principally, even in an institutional setting, differ on the average from other physicians in both their attitudes toward disseminated disease and their approach to the patient and his family.

Their attitudes toward the disease are more objective, yet grasping for every possible hope.

Their approach to the patient and his family is more understanding, yet holding out no false hope.

The physician with greatest empathy, I suppose, would be one who had had cancer himself or still had it.

In November, 1926, Dr. Francis W. Peabody, in a lecture entitled "The Care of the Patient," described the philosophy of medicine which he had pursued as a student, researcher, teacher, administrator, and physician.

Dr. Peabody was professor of medicine at Harvard and director of the Thorndike Memorial Laboratory at the Boston City Hospital.

For him the doctor-patient relationship could be successful only if the doctor was a complete physician, combining human qualities with scientific knowledge and approaching the patient as a total person who happened to be sick.

"What is spoken of as a 'clinical picture,'" Dr. Peabody told students at the Harvard Medical School, "is not just a photograph of a man sick in bed. It is an impressionistic painting of the patient surrounded by his home, his work, his relations, his friends, his joys, sorrows, hopes and fears. . . . Thus the physician who attempts to take care of a patient while he neglects this [emotional] factor is as unscientific as the investigator who neglects to control all the conditions that may

affect his experiment. . . . Treatment of disease immediately takes its proper place in the larger problem of
the care of the patient. . . . The treatment of a disease
may be entirely impersonal; the care of the patient must
be completely personal. . . . One of the essential qualities
of the clinician is interest in humanity, for the secret of
the care of the patient is in caring for the patient.''

It is interesting, perhaps even significant, that Dr.
Peabody should have put together his thoughts and
feelings on the care of the patient, and expressed them
publicly, after he knew that he had cancer.

Less than a year following his lecture and its subsequent publication in JAMA, at the prime of his life and
medical career, Dr. Peabody, aged 46, was dead from his
malignant disease.

3

Responses of Professional Colleagues and Co-workers to a Physician with Cancer

Since the diagnosis of my disease, I have heard from fellow physicians coast-to-coast, graduates of the UB Medical School over a span of 60 years—from 1913 to 1973—representing a variety of disciplines.

Messages have come by word of mouth, by telephone and by letter.

They have reinforced my morale.

I am now—18 months after the diagnosis of disseminated reticulum cell sarcoma and the onset of therapy—psychologically adjusted to my disease and its treatment. I am physically fairly comfortable and leading a satisfyingly active life intellectually and socially.

Yet it is good to hear from old friends and former students, to know that they are thinking of me, that I am not forgotten.

Among the letters that I received was one from a physician and his wife, a registered nurse. Both had been students of mine in pathology 25-30 years ago.

In their letter they speculated that we might all be better health practitioners if, as students, we had experienced the many illnesses we would later have to diagnose and treat in our patients.

As a teacher in medicine, nursing and medical technology, I, too, have toyed with the thought that such a "learning experience" would aid in the development of highly empathic physicians, nurses and technologists.

It is, of course, impossible to include such a "learning experience" in the medical curriculum.

Some clinical conditions are not anatomically and physiologically feasible for both sexes. The male medical student could never experience pregnancy and labor or the female student enlargement of the prostate.

Just running through those that are feasible would delay the practice of medicine indefinitely. Students would be so busy being patients that they would never have time to become medical practitioners. Then we would really have a serious shortage of physicians.

Nor would such a "learning experience" really accomplish its purpose.

If our students were to live to be graduated, all of the diseases they experienced would have to be completely resolvable by themselves or curable, preferably by medical means, without sequelae.

This might give students more empathy with patients undergoing tension headache, URI, impacted cerumen and basal cell carcinoma, but it wouldn't help them empathize with patients suffering from a potentially fatal disease like disseminated cancer.

Such empathy couldn't be acquired by subjecting themselves to a "learning experience" for which they were guaranteed a magical recovery or cure not available to everyone else. (What about students experiencing diagnostic procedures, like sigmoidoscopy, needle biopsy of the liver, etc., which they will order or do on their future patients?)

There are, however, ways in which medical students might learn more than they now do about the physical, psychologic, social and economic problems faced by patients with chronic "incurable" diseases, including disseminated cancer.

They could read—along with their scientific text books, journals, atlases and laboratory manuals—some of the general literature (fiction, poetry, autobiography, etc.) written by and about chronic "incurable" patients over the years.

And is it too far-fetched to suggest that they might attend lectures or discussions at which they could hear and question a guest faculty of physicians, medical students, nurses and lay persons who have themselves had to meet, as best they could, the problems of chronic "incurable" disease?

What has my own "learning experience" taught me about how to respond to another patient—particularly a professional colleague—with disseminated cancer?

On the basis of that experience, and contacts with other physician-patients, I have formulated a list of "woulds" and "would nots." Here are five from that list.

—I WOULD keep in touch with him, particularly during critical periods of his illness.

—I WOULD NOT necessarily express my assurance and good wishes in the conventional ways that symbolize remembrance to a patient spending five to ten days in the hospital with a recoverable, controllable, curable disease.

—I WOULD determine whether he welcomes the opportunity to discuss his disease and its treatment and, if so, discuss them with him.

—I WOULD NOT overlook or minimize his symptomatic or physical state and assume—or pretend—that everything is the same as it was before his diagnosis and treatment.

—I WOULD guard against revealing undue pessimism or offering extravagant optimism on prognosis.

As to "keeping in touch."

In my own case, the most critical period to date was the first three months after diagnosis of disseminated reticulum cell sarcoma and the onset of treatment.

My major battle was a mental and emotional one and I needed all of the support I could get.

I'm sure that support is equally necessary and appreciated in at least two other critical periods—when disseminated cancer turns resistant to available types of therapy, becomes progressive and recurring and, finally, when it lapses into a terminal stage.

The patient with disseminated cancer who is psychologically adjusted and physically comfortable, who can do some work and carry on familial, social and community activities, has less—or no—need for special attention.

His friends will sense his self-reliance and independence.

It was interesting to me how the professional colleagues and co-workers who sustained me during those critical first three months sensed when I began to take hold of myself. When I reached the point where I could go it more or less alone, they stepped out of the picture and let me do so. I am sure, if I need them again, they will be there.

I must say here that there are certain patients who never adjust psychologically to their disease and its treatment, even when their cancer is under therapeutic control or carries a favorable prognosis.

Some openly reject the persons who try to keep in touch with them.

Others accept the attention but are so bitter and resentful that they make their friends feel guilty for being healthy.

I think of a respected physician in his late 50s. Before his illness he was an easygoing, genial fellow, the life of the 10 AM staff gatherings in the hospital coffee shop, the source of most of the humor and the best of the repartee.

His whole personality and behavior have changed since his diagnosis and treatment for carcinoma of the prostate with bony metastases, though the disease is still under symptomatic control after orchiectomy and with hormonal therapy.

He is sullen and unpleasant. He repulses the overtures of professional colleagues and co-workers, even those closest to him.

Gradually they are giving up on him. They have their own problems and responsibilities. Their time is limited, as is the fund of emotion they have to dispense.

They are concluding, one after the other, that in this fast-moving world their time and emotion are best spent on those who need and welcome such expenditure.

As to ways of expressing assurance.

I would consider the needs of the patient.

The short-term hospital patient with a recoverable, controllable, curable disease can usually look forward to a full, normal life.

A patient with disseminated cancer has a chronic, lingering illness. He may be homebound, even confined to a bed or wheelchair. He knows he is facing death. He is liable to feel isolated, lonely, self-absorbed and depressed at times.

Let me illustrate the point I am trying to make by referring to the commonest ways of expressing assurance—flowers, greeting cards and visits.

The bouquet of freshly-cut flowers will cheer the disseminated cancer patient as it does the short-term hospital patient, but only for a brief time.

It lasts just a few days. Watching the flowers wither and die may even remind an introspective cancer patient, with a bent toward thinking symbolically, of his own mortality.

A plant, a terrarium or a dish garden, on the other hand, will last indefinitely, signifying persistent survival. It symbolizes remembrance over a long period.

Tending it, watching it grow, the patient sees it as a friend. He is drawn out of himself. The continuing life of the plant cheers him, gives him a more optimistic outlook on his own life.

So, too, the greeting card that bids the short-term patient "have a speedy recovery" or cracks wise about illness is obviously inappropriate for the patient who is never going to get well.

And the verses and sentiments on cards designed specifically for the "incurable" are often enough to plunge such a patient into a deeper depression than that which he has yet experienced.

But why send a card at all? There are other ways to get a message of assurance over.

A letter or note will serve. It need not be a lengthy one on formal stationery. Indeed a couple of sentences of remembrance and encouragement can be written on a prescription blank.

A postcard sent from a trip to an out-of-town meeting brings the world of medicine closer, for a moment, to the patient who can no longer participate actively in it. So does a copy of the monthly newsletter of the hospital where he had been a staff member or a clipping from a newspaper or medical journal on some topic of interest to him.

In visiting a chronic cancer patient, particularly in a critical period, you have to play it by ear or take a cue from his wife. There are times when he will want you to stick around, when he'll want to hold on to your company.

Other times, when he is having symptoms from his disease or side-effects from his treatment, a visit must be brief. (Toward the end the patient may choose to see only those closest to him.)

If it is impossible to find time to visit him in person, he—or his wife, who needs support too—will welcome a telephone call.

It is important not to promise offhandedly a visit or a phone call and then fail to make it. Anticipation that is not fulfilled may add "disappointment" to the patient's depressive feelings.

A husband and wife, both physicians, have exemplified to me the best possible course for dealing with a professional colleague and friend with disseminated cancer and the side effects of treatment.

As soon as they learned of my diagnosis, they got in touch with me and kept in touch frequently through those critical first three months.

They phoned me or my wife regularly. They were always solicitous and reasonably hopeful.

When they went out of town they sent me postcards.

They have a farm where they spend their weekends. Each Sunday evening, on their way home, they stopped for a few minutes to talk of what had been happening and to leave gifts of their homegrown produce— cucumbers, squash, zucchini, tomatoes. A large, expensive bouquet of long-stemmed American Beauty roses wouldn't have meant so much.

As I improved psychologically and physically, their visits and calls were less frequent, but they still kept in touch.

Parenthetically—while on the subject of ways of expressing assurance—professional colleagues in general seemed less attuned to my mental and emotional needs during those critical first three months than did my co-workers in nursing, social service, medical technology and medical illustration and photography.

A social worker in the cancer institute, a woman with a medical background who, some years ago, had audited my lectures in sophomore pathology, accidentally discovered that I was a patient. Unknown to me she kept a record of my appointments in the lymphoma-leukemia clinic. Whenever I went in, she would "just happen" to run into me and we would talk for ten or fifteen minutes. Those seemingly "chance encounters" were very supportive to me.

The president of the local association of medical technologists called on me at home during the early course of my disease, bringing a message and a remembrance on behalf of herself and the membership.

How often, I wonder, do medical groups take official cognizance of a member with a chronic, long-term, confining, incapacitating, debilitating, potentially fatal illness?

As to discussions and conversations.

Some physician-patients with disseminated cancer, I have found, want to talk openly about their disease with

45

their professional colleagues. They feel frustrated when a visitor skirts the subject, talking of everything else instead.

This is not true of all patients. One physician I knew would burst into tears whenever the word "cancer" was brought up in his presence, even if no reference was made to his own condition.

On the other hand, I personally welcomed the opportunity to discuss my disease and its treatment openly and frankly with my fellow physicians. (Perhaps it was the medical teacher in me coming out.)

Discussion of my experiences was a catharsis. It helped me accept the reality of my plight and made adjustment easier.

Yet hardly any of my professional colleagues ever broached the subject of my disease during our conversations in visits at my home or when we ran into each other outside.

If I raised the subject myself, I could see that it made some uncomfortable, ill at ease. They quickly changed the subject or direction of the conversation. If they did mention my illness, they resorted to euphemisms rather than calling it by its name, "cancer," or "reticulum cell sarcoma."

Even after I had become somewhat adjusted psychologically, the evasive, euphemistic responses of my colleagues bothered me.

They nullified the purpose of our conversations. Instead of bringing us together, those conversations left me feeling not only isolated but also alienated from the person who was talking to me. It was as if there was a glass curtain between us.

Inwardly I found myself sympathizing with professional colleagues as I noted their difficulties in sympathizing with me outwardly.

Sometimes it worried me that they seemed more scared than I was. Could it be, I wondered, that they knew something I didn't know about my diagnosis and prognosis—something from which they were trying to protect me by their silence?

Four examples will illustrate what I mean.

—One colleague of long standing with whom I had always had a close relationship came up to my wife and me at a public dinner. He chatted with her for several minutes, never acknowledging my presence. To him, I thought, I am already a ghost. (And I wasn't being paranoid.)

—One physician on a visit to my home talked to me for half an hour about everything except my disease. Then, when I left the room but was not out of earshot, he questioned my wife sotto voce about all of the things he had been afraid to ask me.

—One morning while waiting my turn for a checkup at the cancer institute I recognized in the corridor an out-of-town physician whom I had known for years. I went up to him and inquired what he was doing there. He had brought in a patient for consultation, he replied. He didn't ask why I was there but, assuming that he might be curious, I told him.

"Yeah, yeah," he muttered. "I heard some time ago that you had a problem." And without adding more he reverted to talking about his patient.

—Another physician, when I told him of my diagnosis, subjected me to a careful clinical history. Then, on

47

leaving, he said: "That's it. That's all. This is the last time I'll ever mention your condition to you."

From a conversational standpoint, the best thing that happened to me during the early months of my disease was developing shingles.

Here was something professional colleagues and co-workers, as well as lay persons, could converse about freely, relate to, identify with. They had no inhibitions, embarrassment or aversion. Indeed, they seemed eager to discuss the subject, relaxed about it.

For my shingles, they gave me the empathy and assurance they couldn't express for my cancer.

As to gauging the patient's symptomatic and physical state.

It's easy for a healthy, active professional colleague to overlook or minimize that state.

How a patient responds to a colleague's attentions will often depend on how he is feeling or looking at the time.

If his response is less than enthusiastic, that doesn't mean that it will always be.

In my own case, I suspect that I lost friends, during the first three months after my diagnosis and onset of treatment, by my refusal of luncheon and dinner invitations.

In the American culture, one of the ways to show attention, goodwill or kindness is to invite someone to eat with you.

On the surface, such an invitation is a good idea for the patient with disseminated cancer who needs to get out and see other people, to get his mind off his own problems.

But radiation and chemotherapy may produce a variety of side-effects. They should be taken into account by the person who proffers a luncheon or dinner invitation.

For three weeks during radiation treatment, because of painful dysphagia from pharyngitis, I lived on macaroni and milk. I had a dry mouth, loss and perversion of taste. I was constantly nauseated. Food was my least concern. I just could not have savored a lavish gourmet meal preceded by cocktails. (Incidentally, alcohol may be a social lubricant but physically it is not an emollient for radiation pharyngitis.)

Certain of the luncheon-dinner invitations from professional colleagues that I declined during those weeks were never repeated. Those who had made them obviously did not understand the reason for my declining their invitations and were hurt because I did so. (Their attitude prompted remorse on my part, further contributing to my psychological difficulties.)

Such lack of understanding was compounded in some colleagues by their obviously hyperbolic cheerfulness about my general symptomatic and physical state.

"Boy, do you look great!" one physician exclaimed boisterously, slapping me on the back.

I had lost about 15 pounds in three weeks under radiation therapy. I was still wearing a shirt with a size 17 collar on a neck that a size 16 might have fitted loosely. The posterior part of my scalp exposed a saucer-sized irregular area of alopecia. My hemoglobin had dropped from 15 to 11 grams and my hematocrit from 49 to 35. When I looked in the mirror before starting to shave in the morning I saw a face that could have served as a model for the tragic side of the mask of Drama.

"What do you say to someone like that?" I asked another patient with active recurring lymphoma of 11 years duration, a man who was under continuing chemotherapy with constant side effects.

The patient, who before his illness had been an administrator in a school of medicine, answered:

"Outwardly I accept the remark graciously and gratefully. But inside myself I think bitterly, 'I only wish I felt that great.'"

A recent report noted that cancer patients "loathed being told by families and friends how well they were looking when they knew they were looking and feeling bad."

As to revealing in any way, even unconsciously, attitudes on prognosis.

I would not add to a physician-patient's burden by undue pessimism (some M.D.s, particularly when a colleague is concerned, just naturally equate cancer with "that's the end") nor would I offend his intelligence with extravagant optimism.

Unless his disease is therapy-resistant or terminal, the average physician with disseminated cancer clings to what hope—however tenuous—there is for control rather than cure of his type of lesion, just as other patients do. (The sick physician is first of all a patient.)

But because of his scientific training and background,

he knows better than they do (if he's thinking straight) how serious his disease is and cannot be fooled by breezy overstatement of hope.

A physician-patient reacts not only to what his professional colleagues (including those taking care of him) say about prognosis but how they say it. He finds clues in their facial expressions, vocal inflections, pauses and interruptions in conversation, physical gestures. Even when he is reasonably well-adjusted, he is vulnerable to any indication of hopelessness.

I still remember three instances from the early months of my illness.

—A physician whom I met on the street spoke of everything but my diagnosis. Then, in parting, he clasped my hand tightly. Solemn-faced, he softly bade me, "Good luck, take care."

—Another physician telephoned me after learning about my reticulum cell sarcoma. He asked how I was feeling. When I replied automatically, in the socially-expected manner, "Fine," he paused perceptibly. Then, with what seemed to me a note of surprise and skepticism, he exclaimed, "Really!"

—And there was the pathologist who interrupted our matter-of-fact conversation about my condition to ask abruptly, in his best "mortality-review" manner, "By the way, Sam, how old are you now?"

Extravagant, breezy optimism on prognosis can be just as bad as, if not worse than, undue pessimism since it assumes that the patient is not really too bright and can be fooled.

About ten days after my first biopsy, an internist who knew of my diagnosis came up to me in the hospital corridor. I had just had my sutures removed and was on my way to pay a social visit to the pathology department. I was yet to be checked for the extent of my disease upon which treatment and prognosis would depend.

"Reticulum cell sarcoma—nothing to worry about," the internist told me confidently. "A few shots of X-ray and you'll be home free. I have several patients with reticulum cell sarcoma who are doing fine. They have never required drugs. In fact, one young fellow who was diagnosed about 15 years ago has gone all this time without any treatment and is still playing tennis." (My first thought, as a pathologist, though retired, was "I'd like to review the slides.")

Eight months later I met the same internist in the same corridor. And I learned that breezy optimism was his approach to disease in others—not in himself.

This time he was so preoccupied that he almost didn't see me. When he did, he made only the most superficial inquiry about how I was doing before blurting out:

"I'm on my way to the pathology department to find out the result on a specimen I left there. Two days ago a dermatologist removed a small brown lesion from the skin of my left temple. He's considering 'cancer' as a possible diagnosis. Believe me, I'm scared to death. I want to get the pathologist's opinion as soon as possible."

That he did—and the opinion of two other pathologists as well.

Their diagnosis was unanimous: "Pigmented seborrheic keratosis —benign."

I shall always remember with gratitude and affection all of the professional colleagues and co-workers who have responded to me in any way during the year-and-a-half course of my disease. (For those in examples I've cited, I fully understand the mental and emotional obstacles which blocked their relating to me freely and easily, openly and frankly. Some, I'm sure, were caught between their desire to comfort and the fear of causing hurt.)

Let me tell you specifically about four colleagues whose attentions were particularly helpful during the critical first three months after my diagnosis and the onset of radiation treatment.

Each had a distinctive professional relationship to me. They were:

—An 83-year-old gastroenterologist who had been my teacher in medical school and with whom I had maintained a friendship for 45 years.

—A 68-year-old out-of-Buffalo surgeon who had been my resident in gynecology when I was an intern.

—A 41-year-old pathologist who had served his residency in the department of which I was a director and had subsequently been associated with me in practice and teaching.

—A 25-year-old intern who had been a sophomore student in my laboratory section the year I retired from UB's department of pathology.

The gastroenterologist, with health problems of his own, was unable to visit me personally because he had given up driving an automobile. He telephoned me immediately after he learned of my diagnosis. From

53

then on he called me or my wife two or three times a week with words of encouragement.

He informed me of patients with a similar diagnosis who were responding to treatment. He kept alive my interest in medicine by asking my opinion on patients whom he was seeing, by quizzing me on material from the medical literature he had read, by seeking my impressions on matters of medical interest in the daily newspaper.

The out-of-town surgeon, suffering from a serious brain lesion himself, wrote regular letters in a shaky script, telephoned long distance when he could no longer write legibly and once came to see me, accompanied by his wife, driven by a university student whom he had employed as a chauffeur.

We had an agreement that if I came across reports of anything new concerning his disease I would let him know immediately and he would do the same for me. We argued about our prognoses. He maintained that disseminated reticulum cell sarcoma—because of the availability of radiation treatment, chemotherapy and immunotherapy—had a chance for a better outcome than the lesion which afflicted him.

He died several weeks after a craniotomy from which he never rallied.

The pathologist telephoned regularly, dropped in unannounced for brief visits and occasionally came to spend the evening. In the three months after diagnosis and onset of treatment, he was the only personal link I had with what had been my professional world for 42 years.

The intern is himself a patient with Hodgkin's Disease, which was diagnosed when he was a sophomore student in the last laboratory section I taught before retirement. He told me about his disease at that time and I visited him when he was hospitalized for a staging laparotomy and splenectomy.

With his disease under control, he finished medical school, was graduated and took an internship outside of Buffalo.

Somehow he heard about my diagnosis of disseminated reticulum cell sarcoma and wrote me in May, 1973. (I have also received mail from him since then.)

Each word, coming from a former student who had been through it all himself—diagnosis, treatment, side effects, psychologic struggle—was loaded for me with empathy and assurance. He wrote:

"Dear Dr. Sanes:

"I have heard through the medical grapevine of your illness and can't tell you what shocking news that was to me. To be faced with malignancy is never an easy experience, but to have this burden so soon after starting a 'new' life makes matters so much more difficult.

"I have felt the fear and frustration that you feel now. I know very well what it is like to wonder what the future will bring.

"I understand that you are responding well to therapy and that chances for cure are excellent. I pray that you will continue to do well and trust that you will return to active life when the stresses of exhausting therapy are no longer there.

"'Carpe diem.' We must learn to appreciate each day and prize each opportunity to enjoy our lives and loved ones.

"Fondest regards to Mrs. Sanes."

4

Relationships with Other Cancer Patients and Some Teachings from Them

Human disease consists of any abnormality in structure and function.

A surgical pathologist diagnoses structural abnormalities in gross specimens and histologic sections.

He seldom, if ever, sees the patient, the living human being—man, woman or child—from whom an organ or part of an organ has been removed.

For example:

A 56-year-old woman with a 2 cm. hard lump in her breast enters the hospital for a biopsy.

From the operating room the excised lump is transported to the surgical pathologist by an OR aide or through a pneumatic tube.

The pathologist examines the lump grossly and reports the microscopic diagnosis of "scirrhous carcinoma" from a cryostat-frozen section by telephone to an OR nurse or through an intercom system to the surgeon.

The patient—a woman with cancer of the breast—
A macro- and microscopic lesion is to him
And she is nothing more.

So cancer was to me as a surgical pathologist. It had to be if I were to perform my specific diagnostic assignment in a scientific, effective way.

But as a surgical pathologist-turned-lymphoma patient I came to see cancer as more than a structural abnormality in a gross specimen and a histologic section.

I also saw it as involvement of the total human being in all of his relatedness to himself, to other persons and to the world about him.

I became keenly aware of the changes that cancer, particularly disseminated cancer, brings about in interpersonal relationships.

The cancer patient relates quite differently from the healthy individual or the one with a benign, temporary illness to his immediate family, more distant relatives, his physician and other members of the medical team, friends and acquaintances among the laity, professional colleagues and co-workers, other cancer patients and the community (in terms of standards and services, institutions and agencies for cancer prevention and care.)

Here are some of the things I have learned as a patient with disseminated cancer through my relationship with other cancer patients during the past two years.

My fellow outpatients at the cancer institute seem surprised to discover that I am a physician. Physicians, in the public's mind, never get sick. At least they never contract the same diseases that other patients do. For example:

One morning in the corridor of the institute I met a lawyer in his late 50s with whom I had worked in community affairs over many years. There was a small dressing on the malar region of his left cheek.

After greeting him, I asked what he was doing at the institute. He replied that he was being treated for basal cell carcinoma.

I told him that I was receiving treatment for disseminated reticulum cell sarcoma.

Noting his puzzlement, I explained that I had "cancer of the lymph nodes."

He was taken aback.

"What!" he exclaimed, looking at me in astonishment and disbelief. "You've got to be kidding! You have cancer? You know—I never before really thought about a doctor getting cancer—being treated for it."

As a physician-patient in the lymphoma-leukemia clinic of the cancer institute, I have found myself a source for information, a partner for scientific discussion, a depository for confidences and a provider of assurance and personal example to other cancer patients.

Hearing me addressed as "Dr. Sanes" by the clinic secretary, nurse, or nurse's aide, some patients ask if I am a medical doctor. Learning that I am, certain of them proceed to put professional questions to me—questions that they say they hesitate to ask the physicians who are looking after them. (Perhaps they are just using me to check on those physicians.)

"How come they didn't do an abdominal operation on me and take my spleen out as they do with other patients?" . . . "Why have they changed my chemotherapy?" . . . "What do they mean I'm in a remission? My lymph nodes are just as large as they ever were." . . . "Did you attend the lecture last week at which that scientist from the National Cancer Institute spoke on the treatment of Hodgkin's Disease? Did he say anything about the drugs I'm on and whether they prolong life? If there's no good evidence that they do, I'm stopping them. The side effects are just too much."

Of course I handle patients' questions gingerly. My suggestion is always, "Why don't you ask your physician? He knows everything about your condition and will be glad to answer you." When possible, I alert the physician to his patient's concerns.

A college English instructor, compelled by his illness to retire, has been disillusioned with me, I'm afraid, as a knowledgeable co-discusser of the scientific aspects of lymphoma-leukemia.

When he found out that I was a physician and a pathologist to boot, he talked to me at length, analytically, about lymphoma-leukemia in general and even individual cell types. He had no qualms about differing with my beliefs and impressions, accumulated over 42 years in pathology.

He spends much of his time reading up on his disease—lymphocytic lymphosarcoma with involvement of peripheral and internal nodes and viscera.

I have a hunch he knows more about the latest medical literature on lymphoma-leukemia than most physicians, even those specializing in the field. Certainly he has read more than I. He can't figure out why I don't read more and he often refers me to the most recent articles. When he has done so, he'll ask me, the next time we meet in the clinic, whether I have read the articles (nearly always I haven't, to his disappointment) and, if so, seek my opinions on the data and conclusions to compare with his.

As to being a depository for confidences, let me cite the middle-aged woman in her 50s who sat next to me one morning in the surgical clinic where I was waiting to have the sutures removed after a third biopsy.

She was reserved and noncommunicative until she heard a nurse address me as "Dr. Sanes." Then her whole manner changed. She confided to me that she had been operated upon a few years previously for cancer of the colon and had returned upon the advice of her family physician for a checkup for possible metastases.

She poured out the most intimate medical and personal details.

"I wouldn't tell these things to any other patient," she explained, "but I know that I can tell them to you because you're a doctor."

(Incidentally, she resided in a small town about 150 miles from Buffalo. Her family physician, who had delivered all her children, had been a classmate of mine in the UB Medical School. I haven't seen him in nearly 40 years.)

The fact that I, a physician, have disseminated lymphoma has seemed to provide a special feeling of assurance, probably even of pride, for other patients with the same disease under similar treatment.

In the first weeks ater my diagnosis, waiting my turn for daily radiation therapy, I overheard an inpatient, a wispy, gray-haired little woman in a pink robe, whisper to another, younger patient from the women's ward:

"Do you see that man over there (indicating me with a nod of her head)? He's a Buffalo doctor. He's got the same disease we have. Getting the same treatment, too."

As a physician-patient, I have felt from the beginning the responsibility to provide assurance and to set an example for other cancer patients by my own reaction to my disease.

Even when I was suffering the darkest fears and the worst side-effects of treatment, once I entered the lymphoma-leukemia clinic I tried to lift my head, throw my shoulders back and walk with an energetic step. When the clinic secretary inquired how I was feeling I'd answer in as firm and resonant a voice as I could muster, so that all of the waiting patients might hear, "Pretty good today."

Learning is a two-way process.

If my fellow patients have learned certain things from me as a physician-patient, I have learned much more from them, not only as a patient but also as a physician.

I have learned from them lessons in some of the fundamental mechanisms for facing and coping with cancer—about the meaning and value of anger, of faith and prayer, of humor and wit, of mutuality.

Anger

Anger is a far commoner emotion among cancer patients than physicians imagine.

It may vary with the presumed origin and cause of the disease, the type, stage, and course.

It may vary with the object against which it is directed, in its intensity and duration, its degree of external expression, and the effects and results it produces.

Because of my scientific knowledge of the etiology and pathogenesis of cancer, I recognized the limits of medicine's understanding of the origin of my disease. I realized that developing "disseminated reticulum cell sarcoma" was just my tough luck. I didn't rail wildly at Fate or God (how come the Devil is never the target?) as patients without my medical training and background often do.

"Why me?" a patient grumbles bitterly. "What did I ever do to deserve this? I've prayed regularly to a beneficent God, whom I always trusted to look after me. Now I have cancer and will probably die of it. I'm still young. My life's goals are nowhere near accomplished. Yet there are men walking the streets in excellent health who have seldom done a virtuous act. Talk about man's abomination to the Lord; what about the Lord's abomination to man?"

In this mood the patient may even decline to have anything to do with a clergyman.

Anger can also be directed against oneself because of feelings of guilt.

—A woman with mammary cancer sees it as her punishment for having refused to breastfeed her children. Another woman with carcinoma of the breast, a topless dancer, attributes it to her "sin" of exposing herself nude in public.

—A physician with advanced cancer of the rectosigmoid berates himself for not having gone in for an examination as soon as the first symptoms appeared.

Some patients vent their anger on a physician, laboratory or hospital. (On occasion, such anger may be patently unfair, unjustified because of the patient's ignorance of the limitations of medical science and practice in regard to cancer at a particular time.)

—A 45-year-old patient who requires treatment for one basal cell cancer of the face after another because he had X-radiation for acne in his teens.

—A middle-aged patient whose physician (a close friend, too, and that may have been the problem) failed for months to take a severe backache seriously enough. He interpreted it as probably due to lumbar osteoarthritis and implied that it might harbor a neurotic or psychosomatic component. Eventually, a diagnostic workup at a medical center to which the patient went in desperation disclosed that the pain was due to multiple myeloma of the spine.

—A physician's wife who requires repeated biopsy for

recurring cancer necessitating surgery. "Why," she mutters rancorously, "should I have to wait a week for a pathology report only to be informed that the biopsy is 'inconclusive' and that another biopsy will be required?"

—A lymphoma patient who absconds from care in a public hospital because the attending staff physician won't talk to him or listen to him about his condition. (On the other hand, a patient may fly into a rage with his physician just for telling him that he has cancer.)

—A woman with a lump in her breast who is told that the necessary biopsy is "not an emergency procedure" and that she will have to wait six weeks for a hospital bed. She had been sold, through public education, on the importance of early diagnosis and prompt treatment for survival in mammary cancer. How should she react but in anger when she reads about the wife of the President of the United States being admitted to a hospital for a biopsy and radical mastectomy the day after discovery of a similar lump?

Pent-up anger can be a sterile, destructive force.

Anger expressed openly, assertively, to a practical purpose, besides acting as an emotional safety valve, can be constructive to the patient's welfare and interests.

The woman who was put off six weeks for a biopsy of a lump in her breast was driven to complain to the editor of the "action" column of her local newspaper. Needless to say she was soon admitted to the hospital.

Anger can be most constructive as a coping mechanism when it is directed against the cancerous disease itself. It can be an antidote for paralyzing fear when it is converted into determination, doggedness, nerve, guts, defiance. "I must go on. I'll beat this son-of-a-bitch of a thing yet." This is an anger bent on life and survival. This is the anger I felt and expressed.

Dr. Robert Cantor of San Francisco, an oncologist who has a degree in psychology, specializes in counseling as well as treating patients with cancer. He has studied 300 of them to find out why some are better able to handle their ailments than others.

He cautions the physician about the patient who takes his disease lightly or passively.

He sees the projection of a patient's anger, even on his family, physicians or nurses ("Just wait, I'll show them all yet!") as a favorable sign.

That patient has a better chance of responding to treatment than one who has nobody to vent his anger on. If, on the other hand, the patient holds his hostility in himself, he is consumed by fear, guilt, depression or unexpressed anger. He will often lose the desire to live or to hang on. Yet, ironically, doctors prefer the nice cooperative patients who are eager to please. . . .

Dr. G. W. Milton of the Melanoma Clinic, Sidney Hospital, Australia, goes so far as to describe "the syndrome of self-willed death" in cancer patients who react without anger.

This syndrome "nearly always affects a big man proud of his virility. The patient, when first confronted with the problem of his malignant disease, appears to disregard it and to be extraordinarily cheerful. To the young doctor

this spurious bonhomie is a matter for great admiration and wonder. . . .
Overnight the patient's whole manner changes and he is physically and mentally transformed. He literally turns his face to the wall and lies inert in bed, covering his face with the bedclothes. . . .
He does not lament his fate nor does he look abjectly miserable. Rather, he gives the impression of being completely indifferent. . . .
Blood pressure, pulse and respiration remain normal. He does not become either cachectic or dehydrated. . . .
Within a month of the onset of this syndrome, the patient will almost certainly be dead. If a necropsy is carried out, although the patient may have an extensive tumor, there will often appear to be no adequate explanation for the cause of death.

"Ire" is what the cancer patient puts into "desire"— the desire to cope with his disease, to survive.

Faith and Prayer

An hour after visiting his semiconscious wife, who had just undergone radical surgery for breast cancer, President Ford addressed 1000 men and women attending a summit conference on the nation's economic crisis.

"It's been a difficult 36 hours," he told them, his jaw working and his voice faltering. "Our faith will sustain us. . . ."

In my adult life, prior to my diagnosis of reticulum cell sarcoma, I had been hospitalized on just four occasions. In each instance I stayed a short time and made a full recovery. During my days in the hospital friends, professional colleagues and co-workers always greeted me jovially with "best wishes."

Since my diagnosis of disseminated cancer I've noticed a change in the tenor of expressions of assurance I receive. Now, most persons quietly offer me their prayers.

Each one of us, when forced to face serious illness, suffering and pain, dying and death, has his own philosophic way of coping whether he has ever verbalized it or not.

In our American culture this way can vary from one based on religion, especially Christianity and Judaism, to a secular one drawn from science and reason. There are all sorts of gradations between.

We derive our philosophic ways of coping from our upbringing, education and personal thinking and experience.

In facing and coping with my own disseminated reticulum cell sarcoma, I have relied on human resources—the knowledge, skill, empathy, and concern of my physicians; physical aid and emotional support from my family and friends; insight, rationality, and adaptiveness on my own part.

At the other extreme, another person in whom cancer is suspected may so trust the divine tenets of his religion and the miraculous power of prayer that he will refuse the promises and ministrations of medical science.

Other patients seek the best of both worlds—the natural or human and the supernatural or divine.

—A middle-aged New York State woman with dis-seminated lymphoma who is being treated at the cancer institute in Buffalo with the latest scientific methods also makes regular trips to Philadelphia for the "laying-on of hands" by a faith healer. She doesn't tell her physicians at the institute about the "second front" attack on her disease.

—A woman in her 60s scheduled for radical mas-tectomy the next morning has her husband telephone to a national "prayer tower" in southwestern United States and ask that it intervene with God for a successful outcome to surgery and cure of her disease.

Interestingly, both patients attribute any favorable results in their condition to faith-healing and prayer, not to their physicians and medical science.

My own philosophic way of coping and that of the other patients mentioned are not typical for most Amer-icans.

More representative is that of a woman in her 50s who has had a personal encounter with disseminated lymphoma. Brought up in a liberal Protestant, non-church-affiliated family, she attended public schools, a state university, and is professionally employed in a field of medical science. By psychologic standards she is mentally and emotionally mature.

"When cancer strikes," she generalizes from her own background, "anger and despair may initially lead a person to deny his religious beliefs, but the rejection is seldom more than temporary.

"The person who has turned to God at other times for lesser reasons will turn to Him again through successive stages of hope if the first one—that the clinical impression be proved wrong by biopsy—is dashed. He'll hope for cure or, if that is not possible, for control and prolongation of life; for palliation and finally for release from agony by death and some type of immortality.

"Certain believers feel a simple, direct, almost childlike closeness to God, such as that of Tevye in *Fiddler on the Roof.* Others approach Him on a more formal, ritualistic level.

"Faith and prayer become increasingly important as their disease worsens, recurs or becomes terminal. Unable to control their situation themselves or to obtain scientific aid and empathy from physicians, deserted emotionally by family and friends, they are led to rely more and more on the spiritual.

"Men and women who have prided themselves on their self-sufficiency are no longer able to go it alone in the face of fear and depression, insomnia, pain, nausea and emesis, loss of weight, debility, cachexia and dehydration and urinary and fecal incontinence.

"Many physicians lack the time, background, training, personality and understanding to give them the presence and support they need. Nor can their families and friends.

"But the cancer patient who believes in God as a loving Father is never alone.

"He is able to talk to God as he cannot talk to his physicians, his dearest friends, the closest members of his family.

"There is comfort for him in the knowledge that he is one of a continuing procession who have called out to God in their time of trouble.

"He can pray with David, 'In thee, O Lord, do I put my trust . . . forsake me not when my strength faileth.' And 'God is our refuge and strength, a very present help in trouble. Therefore we will not fear.' ('Courage,' quotes the Rev. Theodore M. Hesburgh of Notre Dame University, 'is fear that has said its prayers.')

"As a Jew he can look to Job, as a Christian to Jesus, for evidence that suffering and pain are not a symbol of God's rejection.

"And when the battle is finally lost, the believer can hope not only for surcease from suffering and pain but also for survival beyond death. (For some this means a personal, physical resurrection, for others a spiritual reunion with loved ones, for still others genetic and behavioral continuance through their children or historical continuance through remembrance of their thoughts and deeds.)

"He can say, with Paul, 'Death is swallowed up in victory. O death, where is thy sting? O grave, where is thy victory?'

In my own case, I have not so far turned for help to the supernatural.

I have learned, however, that faith and prayer are important coping mechanisms for many cancer patients.

Yet it is not uncommon to hear a physician brand them scornfully as "crutches" for persons too weak to stand alone.

Such physicians do not hesitate to order physically-supportive crutches for the patient with a broken leg.

And they would hail any new safe drug which so influenced a cancer patient's consciousness that he could tolerate his incurable or terminal disease with the same degree of serenity afforded him by faith and prayer. Furthermore, the physician who developed such a drug or proved it by testing would be quick to report it at a national meeting or in a scientific journal. He might even label it a "miracle drug."

Why then scoff at the patient who finds, in the faith of his fathers and through prayer, emotional support, mental uplift and even physical palliation at a time

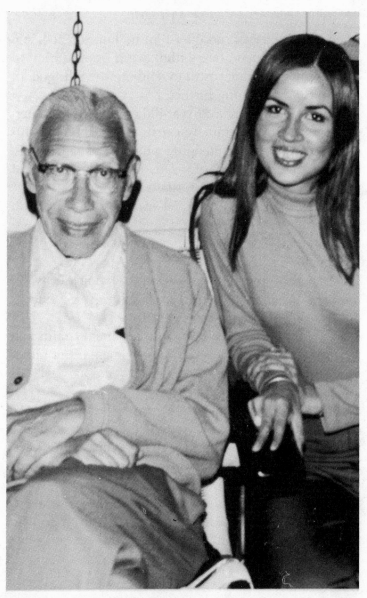

In Guadalajara, Mexico, where he continued to winter until the last year of his illness, Dr. Sanes was cheered by visits from American and Mexican medical students. Here he enjoys a visit with Hilda Margarita Quiroz Galvan, whom he often quizzed about what she was learning.

when his physicians can offer him no hope or help and his family and friends are withdrawing from him?

Even physicians may turn to religion when the gods of science can do nothing further.

Dr. Gary Leinbach, a 39-year-old agnostic gastroenterologist in an academic research institution, lost his scientific objectivity and, doing what any patient might, consulted faith-healers before his death from cancer of the small intestine with metastases.

Some years ago I visited a 50-year-old physician with glioma of the brain whom I had known to be non-observant in religion. I found him reading the New Testament.

"I get comfort from it," he said apologetically. "I thought I had put this stuff aside with my childhood, but somehow it seems to help now."

The wise physician will utilize a patient's faith and prayer as part of his therapeutic armamentarium rather than smile at the sufferer's "simplicity and naivete," his "regression to childhood myths and fantasies."

He can call in a qualified clergyman to assist in the care of the patient, particularly if the patient indicates an interest in religion but has no clergyman of his own. Not all clergymen are qualified. Some, as cancer patients say, "are very good to the sick," but some have the same hangups that physicians and laymen do about cancer and "look with dread upon visits to those who are fighting for their lives against the disease."

Humor and Wit

Cancer is not a matter for levity and flippancy.

Did you ever hear a professional comedian of any

type, even the sadistic Don Rickles, make cancer or the cancer patient the butt of his gags?

Molly McGee of radio's "Fibber McGee and Molly" would have said "T'ain't funny, McGee."

Healthy persons find it hard to take "cancer" as a fun subject.

"All in the Family" once ran a program on the threat of breast cancer and a possible mastectomy for Edith Bunker. Happily, the lesion proved benign. A woman, assumedly not a cancer patient, protested in a letter to the TV editor of *The New York Times*:

"I fail to see how the above-mentioned episode, which dealt with a profoundly disturbing problem could even remotely be called humorous. The fact that the episode . . . happy ending . . . does not absolve its producers from showing greater responsibility and sensitivity. . . ."

An English play, "The National Health," found cancer, among other serious illnesses, a subject for laughter. Clive Barnes, critic for *The New York Times*, labeled the play an exploration "into the queasily dangerous area of bad taste" but felt that the playwright's comedic approach was redeemed by his "compassion and concern. . . ." "He regards life so highly," Barnes wrote, "that he can make a joke about terminal cancer and get away with it."

Cancer patients resent even more than healthy persons do any indication that others take cancer lightly.

"I don't mind joking about my condition," one commented, "provided I do it myself." (Actually, the "All in the Family" program mentioned before was urged upon the producer by a woman aide who had had a mastectomy.)

There is, in fact, a certain amount of good-natured "needling," joshing and banter among physicians and other members of the medical team and their patients in the lymphoma-leukemia clinic in the cancer institute.

Cancer patients with a sense of humor and a knack for wit who joke about other matters are quite capable of doing so about their own disease and themselves. Usually it is a self-kidding, bitter-tender, ironic, sort-of-gallows humor but humor nevertheless.

—Mrs. Birch Bayh, wife of the senator from Indiana, after undergoing a mastectomy for cancer of the breast, referred to herself and fellow patients as "bosom buddies."

—Another woman who had been surgically treated for mammary cancer wrote to Mrs. Ford, wife of the nation's President, an archetypal Republican conservative: "Perhaps we 'radicals' could get together."

—A high school girl with whom I would wait in the hematology OPD clinic "guessed" that she must have caught leukemia from going to the movies too frequently. She saw "Love Story" (in which the heroine had leukemia) five times.

—A teen-aged boy under radiation therapy for Hodgkin's Disease stumped me with the riddle "Why is a patient under radiation treatment like a pornographic movie?"

"I don't know," I responded. "Why?"

"Because they're both X-ra(y)ted. Get it?"

—A college girl composed but didn't submit a three-word, three-line rhyming verse in response to a Buffalo

74

newspaper columnist's invitation to a "shortest poem" competition.

In those three words and three lines her verse was an epic poem, covering the whole struggle for adjustment by the patient discovered to have lymphomia-leukemia.

> "Mope
> Hope
> Cope."

—I visited in the hospital a physician of my age group, a former student of mine and a professional colleague for 37 years, with metastases showing up less than 18 months after the original resection of the colon for cancer. (We had both learned of our diagnoses at the same time in February, 1973.) He had received a course of radiation and was suffering from severe radiation proctitis as well as the side effects of chemotherapy.

He lay in bed, his face creased in pain. I stood at the bedside.

After our initial greeting, we were both silent. Then he looked up at me seriously and said, "Sam, would you do something for me?"

"Anything," I replied, "anything at all. What is it?"

"Will you please find me the name of the guy who coined the term 'the golden years'?"

"But why?"

"I want to give him a good kick in the ass."

"Hoping all the time," I rejoined, "that he also has radiation proctitis."

You should have heard the two of us disseminated cancer patients explode into laughter so loud that it must have startled the patient in the room across the corridor.

—There was nothing laughable to the onlooker in the sallow-faced young woman with dark circles under her eyes who hobbled into the lymphoma-leukemia clinic doubled up in pain. Her husband walked behind her, his arms around her waist, his hands pressing on her abdomen.

A nurse hurried up, offering to bring a wheelchair.

"No," the patient thanked her. "The pain is less when I walk this way. The pressure of my husband's hands seems to relieve it."

"Isn't there something I can do?" the nurse persisted.

"Yes," the patient responded with a wry laugh as she leaned doubled up over the clinic secretary's desk. "How about getting me a 'whole body transplant'? Don't you have a Dr. Frankenstein on your staff?"

—Another woman sat next to me in the diagnostic X-ray department. She had had surgery for cancer of the rectum and had a colostomy, hepatic and pulmonary metastases.

Looking up from the morning newspaper she had been reading, she turned to me and sighed wistfully, "If only one of those 'breakthroughs' I'm always reading about in the headlines would turn out to be a 'true break' for us cancer patients."

Humor, genuinely felt and expressed, is an excellent coping mechanism for some cancer patients. It saves them from denying their predicament, from indulging in self-pity. It releases inner tensions. And it permits them to make other patients as well as themselves feel brighter and better.

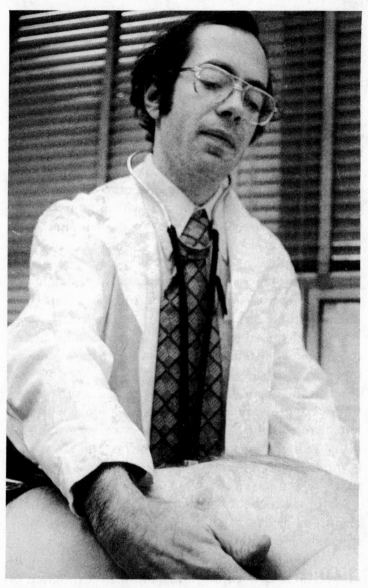

A physical examination was part of Dr. Sanes' biweekly visits to the leukemia-lymphoma clinic at Roswell Park Memorial Institute. Here Dr. Michael C. Snyderman feels for palpable nodes.

Mutuality

Albert Schweitzer wrote of the brotherhood of those who suffer pain.

I write of another brotherhood, perhaps a closer, more exclusive one, that of cancer patients, particularly those with the same type and stage of cancer.

Cancer patients identify with each other in a different, more intimate way than they do with persons among other groups to which they belong, including their immediate families.

For example:

A 50-year-old woman with presumptive carcinoma of the sigmoid was admitted to the colon service of the cancer institute for a resection.

The patients on the floor visited her, included her in the group. They talked to her, told her to have courage, made her feel "one of the family."

When the operation disclosed a benign lesion, everything changed. The other patients still spoke with her, but there was a difference. She was no longer one of them. Politely but firmly they shut her out. (It was an example, you might say, of the "haves" versus the "have nots.")

My own experience and observations bear out what I read in an article, "Cancer Patients Help Themselves," from which I shall borrow certain statements.

The empathy of cancer patients for each other can be of real value as a coping mechanism in a program of treatment and rehabilitation.

For years I have heard lay persons and physicians who haven't had cancer themselves decry the "segregation" of cancer patients in their own clinics and hospitals, groups and clubs and hospices for the dying.

Cancer patients, they have emphasized, are just like any other patients and should be treated as such. It is "unhealthy" to consider them otherwise.

Now, on the basis of my own experience and observations of other patients, I would take some exception to that attitude.

In a hospital where there are no natural, informal, spontaneous groups of certain kinds of cancer patients, it could be valuable to create officially-structured ones.

The association with fellow cancer patients "meets an individual's need for security, belonging, companionship and mutual support" from those like him, a need that can be met in no other way.

Let me give some examples.

The lymphoma-leukemia clinic for adults at the cancer institute is a natural, spontaneous, informal group not only for patients but also for the members of their immediate families who accompany them.

At any morning session where I go for a checkup there are 15-30 patients of all ages, backgrounds, and walks of life. There are others like me. I am not alone.

The clinic group acts as a reinforcement community or group therapy session for both patients and relatives. (It is often difficult to tell from their appearance which is which.)

Long-time patients talk to each other, compare notes on their disease, tests, therapy, and its side effects. They air their worries and concerns, gripes and peeves, problems of everyday living. They also talk about the pleasant happenings and enjoyable activities in their lives.

New patients are "surprised and relieved that others felt helplessness," uncertainty and frustration just as they do. A patient may be calmed by learning that others, too, have thought of suicide as a way out and have managed the situation in their own ways. "I thought I was the only one to ever think of suicide. I thought I was crazy for thinking it."

Within the group praise for psychologic strength and perseverance may help patients renew their feelings of self-esteem.

As the weeks pass, the whole group takes courage from seeing a fellow patient make good progress. Certain patients with five-to-ten-year survival or "cure" prove even the improbable dream comes true.

Sometimes one patient will fail to show up and word will go around that he is worse and has been admitted to the cancer institute as an in-patient. If, in a few weeks, he is back in the clinic again in good spirits, it is evidence that another battle has been won, for a while anyway. If he does not return, some of the group, who have formed a close attachment for him, suffer a wrench.

But they keep on hoping, with trust in their physicians and a long-shot gamble on research. They obtain satisfaction and support from sharing their ability to keep going despite everything.

"How are you this morning?" inquires the clinic secretary of a lymphoma patient on a revisit. "Terrible," answers the woman, "but I'm here and that makes all the difference in the world."

What is true in the outpatient clinic is also true among hospitalized patients. They support each other in times of stress.

A physician who had to undergo radical surgery for infiltrating, recurring but non-metastasizing cancer lay in bed, depressed, refusing to talk to anyone, including his wife.

The woman who occupied the room across the corridor had extensive cancer with no prospects for control and cure. All she could hope for was palliation. Her husband denied the seriousness of her disease and didn't visit her. But she refused to surrender. Getting dressed one morning, she crossed the corridor to say a word to the doctor, whose depression the nurses had told her about.

"Come on," she said. "Get up. Look at all the other patients. Look at me. And you're an M.D. I'm going to the beauty parlor and when I come back I expect to see you up and walking around."

Her efforts, along with those of another patient, a college student with multicentric cancer, finally did what the professionals had been unable to do—got the physician-patient out of bed and onto the road to psychologic adjustment for operation.

During the first three months after my own diagnosis and the onset of radiation therapy, I often fretted about my condition, whether the side effects I was experiencing were real or whether I was neurotically imagining them.

At my lowest ebb, my wife called a friend, a clergyman who had been under treatment at the institute for disseminated reticulum cell sarcoma for ten years. She relayed to me what he told her about his own early reactions to his disease and its treatment, his subsequent progress and setbacks. Aware though I was that every case differs, it was very reassuring to me to know that he had come through it all and was still pursuing a happy, productive life.

A year later I was able to give some of this same reassurance to another physician with disseminated cancer when he was placed on chemotherapy. Alarmed at how he felt, he telephoned me to compare side effects and I could assure him that what was happening to him was perfectly "normal" in relation to the drug he was taking.

Yet despite all the evidence that cancer patients can and do help each other, many physicians are fearful of their "interference" in the treatment and rehabilitation picture.

It is difficult to persuade some physicians to act as sponsors or advisors for groups of cancer patients who have undergone definitive treatment—"laryngectomies," "ostomies," "mastectomies"—and want to band together, in officially organized groups, for mutual comfort and support and to help others.

Sometimes a head of service or an administrator will refuse to permit representatives of such groups to visit patients in the hospital before and after treatment.

I myself was politely turned down by a hospital social worker whom I met at a public function.

"Now that I am doing fairly well myself," I suggested, "I might be able to give some psychologic support to other physicians with disseminated cancer while they are hospitalized. Do you think that you could use me? I would be glad to come in to see them and talk with them."

"Oh, I'm afraid that some attending physicians wouldn't like that," she told me. I heard nothing more of the matter.

Obviously hospital visiting should be done only by persons who are properly qualified, selected, trained and oriented.

The physician should realize, however, that there are things that he and other members of the basic medical team cannot do for certain cancer patients and be prepared to utilize anyone who can help.

The list is a long one. Besides clergymen and other cancer patients, it includes dentists, secretaries, social workers, psychiatric and family counselors, visiting nurses, homemakers, physical and vocational rehabilitation and prosthetic specialists, representatives of the Cancer Society and other community agencies, officials of industry, labor and government.

The coping ability of cancer patients, particularly those active with disseminated disease, in the face of their uncertain future never ceases to impress me.

—I was waiting my turn in the lymphoma-leukemia clinic one day when a new patient came in and sat down beside me. He was obviously frightened. It showed in his eyes, his voice, his posture.

"Your next patient is terribly scared," I told my physician as I went into the examining room.

"They all are," he responded. "The remarkable thing

is how well, in time, they cope, even when they have to be hospitalized. Ninety-five percent of them meet their disease not only with courage and with life-affirming drive but even with heroic efforts to continue their everyday activities. Only five percent give up—lie in bed in a fetal position with eyes tightly shut or the bed-clothes pulled over their heads or sit all day in a chair, glum and silent, guzzling beer."

If ever I start sinking into a slough of discontent and self-pity when doing as well as can be expected with my cancer, I will quickly pull myself up through the lesson I learned from this incident in the lymphoma-leukemia clinic.

—An ambulatory patient with a reputation as a chronic complainer, a man in his 60s, was listing his gripes in a whining voice—gripes about his state of health, his treatment, his personal and family problems. (Actually he was in remission.) A woman patient known for the low boiling point of her temper and for her outspokenness listened as long as she could stand it. Then:

"What are you griping about?" she virtually yelled at the other patient so that everybody could hear. "You're alive, aren't you!"

5

The Effect of Cancer on the Family of the Patient

"I have a question to put to you. Since it is my observation that frequently a family member needs more help than a cancer patient, I wonder why you do not write about this."

The retired public health nurse who made that comment is herself a ten-year survivor with lymphosarcoma, stage III-IV.

She is married and has one son. Her mother and a brother, both still living, have been treated for cancer. Before and after her retirement she had worked with cancer patients and their families professionally and as a volunteer.

Her question, I knew, was based on personal experience and trained observation.

It hit me hard.

How often, I thought, do physicians—healthy themselves and without the experience of cancer in their immediate families—pay more than superficial attention to the family of a cancer patient for whom they have accepted primary responsibility?

In some instances they may not even realize that the patient has a family.

This is true for medical students too.

At the invitation of the chairman of the UB Department of Pathology, I conducted a seminar for the entire sophomore class on "What a Cancer Patient Expects from a Physician."

In how many clinical conferences to date, I asked the students, had they been actually introduced to the family of a patient, its problems, and needs? Not once, they told me, except in a course in genetics, and then for scientific purposes.

I asked the same question of a graduating senior and received the same answer in regard to clinical conferences in the third and fourth years.

Yet there are those who believe that the way a cancer patient, particularly one with advanced, incurable disease, adjusts to his diagnosis, how he accepts treatment, even how long he lives, depends to a certain extent on his relations to family members and their response to him.

The physician who accepts a cancer patient professionally, therefore, has a double responsibility. Primarily he is responsible for the well-being of the affected person but also, in a measure, for that of his family.

In any type and stage of cancer both may need help in coping with the initial psychologic shock and panic induced by the diagnosis.

If the cancer is stage I-II and treatment proves effective, promising long-term survival or "cure," the continuing effects on the family, as on the patient, may be minimal.

But there can be problems even when the outlook

seems to be a favorable one. For some patients and families the treatment and its consequences may be nearly as difficult to accept as advanced, incurable disease. It is not easy to face up to radical mastectomy, colostomy, laryngectomy, radical head and neck surgery, amputation of a limb or operations involving the sex organs.

The major problems, however, come during the treatment and follow-up of patients who fall in the 65-70 percent estimated by the American Cancer Society to have residual, disseminated, therapy-resistant, progressive, recurring, complicated, terminal disease within five years after the original diagnosis and treatment.

The family, like the affected person, is totally unprepared for those problems, as it is for the initial diagnosis.

They are not only physical but mental, emotional, sexual, social, economic, religious, and philosophic ones.

How it meets them may affect not only the patient's condition and course, but the well-being and survival of the family itself.

Cancer in a family may be so divisive and destructive a force that it produces sufficient tension and friction to lead to estrangement, separation, and divorce.

On the other hand, it may be so strengthening and unifying that it leads to a closer, deeper, and more sustaining relationship than ever existed before.

What happens within the family depends not only on its individual members but on the patient's physicians, hospital and other health-care personnel (special therapists, social workers, family counselors, visiting nurses, homemakers, health aides, clergymen); employers, friends and neighbors; other cancer patients and families; the local unit of the American Cancer Society; community facilities and services.

Varied factors cause varying situations in various families.

So the families of cancer patients have problems and may need help.

Let's take two almost completely contrasting examples.

Example I
Family Profile

An 85-year-old retired man lived in a small rural community (population 600). He and his wife, 82, had been married more than 60 years. They had a son who was a physician and two daughters who were professionals in fields allied to medicine. All lived in other parts of the United States.

The man had considered himself to be in good health. Lately he had taken laxatives for constipation. He was mentally and socially alert. He and his wife were self-reliant. They went shopping, did their own housework and outside chores, and took care of a large garden. Their income was limited—Social Security and a small pension—but enough for their needs.

Clinical Condition and Course of Patient

One night, a couple of hours after dinner, the husband was seized with colicky abdominal pain. When it became obvious that there was something wrong and it wasn't going to right itself, the wife called the family doctor. He came to the home and made a presumptive diagnosis of "acute bowel obstruction." He then called the town's volunteer fire department, which dispatched its ambulance to take the patient to a university teaching center hospital 70 miles away.

There, an emergency colostomy was performed about 2 AM for an obstruction of the descending colon from what appeared to be a localized carcinoma.

Two weeks later a resection of the colon with lymph nodes and mesentery was done. There was no gross intraperitoneal-hepatic spread. Pathologic examination showed a highly-differentiated adenocarcinoma, Dukes' A. All nodes were free of cancer. (X-ray films of the chest taken preoperatively were negative for metastases.)

The patient, after an uneventful postoperative course, returned home. He subsequently was readmitted to the hospital for closure of the colostomy. Again there were no postoperative complications. The hospital stay was of normal length.

Regular follow-up examinations have been negative for recurrence, metastases or new primary lesions in the rectum and colon.

One-and-a-half years after resection of the colonic cancer, the patient was in excellent health. He journeyed by car and plane to visit children, cousins, brother, and sister. He walked a mile or so a day, took an active interest in life around him.

Effects on Family

Throughout the husband's and father's illness, family problems were few.

One was the distance of the hospital from the home.

The patient wanted his wife close at hand but daily visits were impossible. They compromised on daily, sometimes twice-a-day, phone calls.

The physician-son, notified by his mother, got in touch with his father's surgeon immediately. The surgeon was happy to keep him informed by long-distance telephone and the son relayed the information to his mother and two sisters.

All three children telephoned their parents regularly— one of the daughters from abroad where she was vacationing.

When the father was finally discharged, the surgeon supplied the son with a full record, including copies of the operative, laboratory, X-ray and pathologic reports.

When the pathologic report verified the diagnosis of cancer, the question arose as to whether the surgeon should tell the patient. He consulted the wife and son. The patient had recently lost a sister and a brother-in-law to cancer. Because of his age, type of personality, and dread of the disease—and because of the clinical and pathologic stage and histologic grade of the lesion—it was decided not to be specific about the findings unless he asked. He did not. He was satisfied with the diagnosis of "tumor."

This posed an additional problem for the wife since a few close friends and relatives knew that the tumor was malignant. Some of them were elderly and she could not be sure that they would not use the word "cancer" inadvertently in talking to the patient. She sat in on all conversations, monitoring them carefully.

After the resection the patient was eager to go home

as soon as possible despite the colostomy. He could not take care of it himself, so the wife called the community health nurse who showed her how to do it.

Concerned about her husband's loss of weight, she prepared tasty, nourishing meals and encouraged him to eat even when he wasn't hungry. She also devised a system of pulleys and ropes by which he could pull himself up in bed and exercise his arms and shoulders during his convalescence.

A devout believer, though not a regular church-goer, the wife found strength in prayer. Friends and neighbors were attentive and helpful.

The illness caused no real financial problems. Medicare, Blue Cross-Blue Shield, and a retiree's extended benefits plan met nearly all of the hospital and medical bills, which amounted to $7210. The most difficult thing for the wife was filling out the numerous complicated forms required for reimbursement and straightening out the inevitable foulups not of her making. Finally, tears running down her cheeks, she sought the assistance of a social worker in the County's Office of the Aging.

The second example was different from the first in nearly every way.

Example II
Family Profile

The patient lived in a suburb of a metropolitan county (population 1,100,000) with his wife of eight-and-a-half years and their two sons, aged 3 and 5. Though only 30, he was already an executive in a firm that did business throughout the state. A promising career lay ahead of him.

His wife, 29, was one of a close family of nine children. Her father, a graduate of the University of Buffalo Medical School, had been a family practitioner prior to his death of coronary heart disease. Her mother was a registered nurse. One brother was a physician, one sister a nurse. An uncle also was a physician, a graduate of the UB Medical School.

The couple had worked together in the same office prior to their marriage and the wife often said that when both children were in elementary school she would like to return to the business world. Meanwhile they shared the responsibilities and decisions for the home and the children.

The husband was an avid golfer, often competing in area tournaments. The wife was learning the game.

They had recently bought their own home and joined a country club.

Clinical Condition and Course of Patient

In early November the husband developed a persistent cough and low-grade fever. His personal physician, a family practitioner, admitted him to a teaching hospital affiliated with a local medical school.

X-ray films of the chest revealed abnormalities. The right testicle was enlarged.

Two days after the patient's admission, a urologist was called in consultation. He recommended an operation. This was delayed for a week because of congestion in the lungs shown on the X-ray films.

The final pathologic diagnosis was returned two days

after orchiectomy. It was "embryonal carcinoma." The next morning the patient was transferred to a cancer institute by ambulance.

There clinical, X-ray and laboratory examinations, and staging procedures showed the carcinoma to be disseminated with retroperitoneal, mediastinal and pulmonary metastases.

Experimental chemotherapy, including bleomycin, was prescribed, to be given in courses.

The side effects during the first course were severe. The patient suffered gastric hemorrhaging and had to be fed through a nasogastric tube and intravenously. For several days he was on the critical list. In subsequent courses of chemotherapy the side effects were milder. The patient was weak and tired. He didn't eat and lost weight. He lost some of the hair on his head.

A week after his admission to the institute the patient was given a pass to spend Thanksgiving Day with his family.

He was discharged as an inpatient a few days before Christmas. Metastases had diminished in size with chemotherapy. He would continue with weekly visits as an outpatient.

After two weeks at home he returned to his employment on a part-time basis but was soon working full time. He felt relatively well.

He was readmitted to the institute on March 2 for a surgical approach to removal of the remaining metastases in the abdomen and chest.

The operation was performed the next day but the disease had spread too far to be eradicated by surgery. The patient didn't rally from pulmonary complications (fibrosis, embolism, and anoxia) and hepatic and renal necrosis, apparently of anoxic origin.

After a little more than two weeks in the intensive care unit he was transferred to another hospital for support of his vital functions by machines. Most of the time he was unconscious. Death came three days later, March 22.

Effects on Family

From the moment of the first hospitalization the husband and wife shared their fears and hopes. They talked freely, participated in making decisions.

The most frustrating period for both was the 12 days in the first hospital. The family physician saw the patient every day but was noncommittal. He never talked with the wife. She tried desperately to get to see him and talk with him. She telephoned his office. His secretary assured her that he would call her back. He didn't. She spoke to the hospital receptionist and left a message for the doctor when he signed in, asking him to come to her husband's room to talk to her. He didn't. Thinking he might not be in the hospital afternoons and evenings when she usually visited, she made it a point to go in twice in the morning. Perhaps, she thought, she could see him when he was making rounds. The nurse told her that he had already left.

As the days passed, the wife's anger and bitterness grew. She had the feeling that the physician was avoiding her. She resented not knowing what was going on. What did the X-ray films show? What was the outlook?

The urologist was more open and informative. The husband and wife both liked him.

When the pathologic report was in, he went to the husband's room at 6 PM and told him that the tissue in the resected testicle was malignant and that there were a few spots on his chest film that were not due to pneumonia but cancer. He would be transferred to the cancer institute the following morning. "They know all about it."

When the wife came in at 7 PM the husband didn't greet her with his usual smile. He had always been able to cover up pain and fear. Now, however, he "cried like a baby" as he told her that he had cancer, that it had already spread, that he was being transferred to the cancer institute.

He was going to die, he knew. Only a year before he had watched two of his "buddies" in their 30s die of malignant disease at the institute.

The wife didn't cry—not then. She sat on his bed, her arms around him, telling him that he must hope, that he didn't have to die.

She cried later, in the car driving home. She continued to cry softly, so that the children wouldn't hear her, after she went to bed. Although she was exhausted, she couldn't sleep. She cried most of the night.

The next day she had the problem of telling the children, her husband's family, her own, both out of town, and his close friends and co-workers.

She told the children only that their father was seriously ill and would have to be in the hospital for some time. She feared that if she used the word "cancer" some playmate to whom they repeated it might tell them that cancer was a fatal disease, that their father was going to die. As it was, they weren't really frightened. The younger boy had been hospitalized shortly before. He had come home. There was no reason to suspect that his father might not.

Both her own family and her husband's reacted with love and concern and were supportive throughout the husband's illness.

Neither her mother nor her brother, however, was optimistic about the outcome. They knew too much about the disease.

The sister who was a nurse in a pediatric intensive care unit on the West Coast was more comforting. Later, during the final stage of the husband's illness, she flew East to "special" him and console her sister.

The husband's mother met the news with optimism, sending word to her son that he "mustn't give up." His father said little.

Friends and neighbors tried to buoy up the wife's spirits. She found hope in the fact that one of the neighbors, an elderly man, was doing well under treatment for incurable cancer, the disease apparently in remission.

At the institute there was no further problem of "not knowing" what was going on.

The wife had an obsession to know everything, the bad as well as the good.

She had not mentioned at the first hospital that she was from a medical family and she did not do so at the institute until the end, after her husband's surgery.

But on the morning of his admission a physician took both husband and wife to the solarium and gave them a forthright account of what to expect. He answered all questions.

He told them that he could make no definite prognosis, but that the average the husband could expect to live without treatment would be three months.

There was no definitive treatment. Chemotherapy and surgery were being employed experimentally. There could be serious side effects to the chemotherapy. There was no certainty that anything that could be done would change the three-month average.

The couple talked it over and decided to take the gamble.

When the physician left them alone, the wife asked her husband if he would have made the same decision were he a bachelor.

He admitted that he probably would not have risked the side effects for such uncertain benefit if he had not had a wife and children.

Throughout his hospitalization there was no attempt to conceal from him or his wife anything about his condition.

The physician gave the husband permission to pull his own chart at the nurse's station. He did so, pointing out to his wife what it said about his condition.

The head of service made it a point to see the wife when he made his rounds. If she was not in her husband's room, he sent someone to find her or if she had gone home called her on the phone. He gave her other numbers besides his office where he might be reached at any time—the institute library, his home.

After her husband's surgery, when she was spending up to 24 hours a day at his side, a medical social worker sought her out and asked if there was anything she could do to help. She offered her a locker to keep her things in, showed her how to get to the cafeteria, volunteered to help her find a place to stay near the institute. Although the wife never had to call upon her for anything more, she was most grateful.

After the first shock of the diagnosis of disseminated, metastatic cancer, the husband and wife kept up each other's spirits with hope, understanding, even humor.

The husband looked and felt awful during the courses of chemotherapy. But if his wife, watching him, let her concern show on her face he would chide her.

"Don't start moping," he admonished her once, "If you do, no matter how I feel, I'm going to get out of bed and give you a great kick in your you-know-where."

It worked. Later, after he had died, the wife said that she had never been really depressed—fearful and lonely, but not depressed. When her husband was on the critical list during the first course of chemotherapy she cried, but out of sheer fright. Until the end she kept up her spirits, her will to fight.

"Others had told me how depressed they were when a loved one had cancer," she recalled. "Sometimes I'd wake up in the morning and think, 'Is this the day I'm going to be depressed?' I never was. I told myself it was going to be a long battle but we'd make it. I took it day by day, thanking God as each day passed."

She did sometimes feel "boxed in" sitting for long hours at her husband's bedside. Things seemed to be closing in on her. At such times, her husband would urge her to get out, to go shopping. If friends dropped in he would ask them to take her out for dinner and a drink.

She was torn between her desire to be with her

husband, to give him all of her time, and her duty to her children. Neighbors and friends looked after them. A younger sister came to stay for a while. When it became obvious that the end was near she sent them to her mother in another city where they would feel secure and loved. But she missed them when she returned briefly to the dark, empty house. Often when she did so she fell into bed too physically and emotionally exhausted to even take off her clothes.

Although there were times when her husband didn't want her or anyone else to see him, they were few. He wanted to spend as much time as possible with her though he talked, she said, mainly of his work.

On Thanksgiving Day, when he had not seen his children for nearly three weeks, he asked for and received a pass to leave the institute. His sister and brother-in-law, who lived nearby, invited the family to their apartment so that he would not have to travel to his own more distant home. But when he got there he had no appetite for food, company or activity. He was sick and tired, happy to just lie on the couch. They took him back to the institute early.

Both husband and wife had been brought up in devout Catholic homes. The husband had for a time been a seminary student. But in later years he had thought less of the rituals of religion. Sunday had become a day for playing with the children and golfing rather than going to church.

In the institute, a young priest visited him for long talks which brought him much peace of mind. He attended Mass. His parents, particularly his mother, rejoiced when he told them. (Ironically the priest who had been so helpful left the priesthood shortly before the patient died.)

The priest never looked up the wife, but after her husband entered the institute she found that it gave her peace and comfort to go to a nearby church and just sit quietly there, away from the immediacy of the institute, praying. She did not attend regular services and neither saw nor asked to see a priest.

She asked questions of God, not in anger but in puzzlement. Why should her husband have cancer? Why should he be facing death? Why should the children lose a father? There was no answer. She has not yet, she says, been able to accept the dictum, "Thy will be done," but hopes to some day.

The two months at home, between the husband's December discharge from the institute and his readmission in March for surgery, were bitter-sweet, a blend of happiness and sadness.

"What a miracle!" the wife wrote to friends who had left town for the winter. "Only eight weeks ago he was so very sick and now he is thoroughly enjoying every minute of every day."

Not, perhaps, "every minute." The husband realized that his improvement might be only temporary. He took his insurance policies out of his safe-deposit box and left them with his insurance agent where they would be readily available. The box would be inaccessible after his death.

The children were taken care of financially, but the husband wished now that he had spent more time with them, less on the golf course. If his improvement continued, he said, they would take a trip with the children.

With cancer and treatment he had become impotent. "It doesn't matter," the wife assured him. "I'm so glad to have you here, alive and better. That's all I care about."

Before his illness they had slept in twin beds. When he came home after the institution of chemotherapy, they shared a double one. He felt better close to her. Often they would go to bed at 9:30 and talk until midnight.

The children delighted in having their father home again. At Christmas they helped him dress as Santa Claus for an office party, gave him a hat to cover his thinning hair.

They seemed to understand that they couldn't run into the bedroom as they had once done in the morning, to waken him with kisses and roughhousing. Instead they cuddled close and played quiet games with him.

Returning to work part time, then full time, he made few concessions to his disease.

A friend gave him a wig that he wore jauntily, making no pretense that it was his own hair, taking it off for laughs.

When four old friends dropped in weekly to visit, they all drank beer together, though he had to excuse himself and go to the bathroom to throw up every 20 minutes.

He went back to the institute for surgery, still optimistic that somehow by some miracle he would yet be cured.

After the operation, the institute bent its rules for

visiting in the intensive care unit so that the wife could stay with him around the clock. When his sister-in-law flew in, she was given permission to "special" him so that the wife could get some rest.

The physician kept her informed about what was going on.

Once, while sitting at her husband's side after the operation, she broke down and cried, thinking he was asleep. He opened his eyes, pressed her hand, and summoned enough strength to wink at her. Soon after, he sank into a coma and never regained consciousness.

After his death, the wife told the children that their father had gone to Heaven. Both she and he had believed in personal immortality.

"I don't want my daddy to die," the little one protested, weeping stormily.

The older one was calmer. He hugged his mother, told her not to cry. Later he told his little brother that he, too, had wanted to cry, "but if I did, that would only make mommy cry more."

Because the husband was on experimental therapy, there was no charge for his treatment at the institute. But the bill for the initial hospitalization and physicians totaled $2172, that for the final three days in the second hospital $8410. Insurance took care of almost all of the expenses. Throughout the husband's illness, his employer paid full salary and insurance premiums.

In the days that followed the mother talked often with the little boys about their father, recalling the happy times. She was honest with them. She told them that their father had died of cancer, that all that could be done for him had been done, but that the disease had been discovered too late to be cured.

They were curious about the Heaven where he had gone.

"Do they have birthday cakes there?" the little one asked one day.

Today the wife is working part time when the children are in school.

Family and friends give her love and encouragement, but it is a lonely life despite them. At night, when the children have gone to bed, there is no one to talk to, to plan with, to love.

She dreams, all over again, that he has cancer. Once she awakened at 3 AM and couldn't go back to sleep, thinking of her husband and their life together.

She got out of bed, found the movie projector and some old home movies. Alone in the darkness she watched her husband and herself in happier days playing with the children.

Then, comforted, she went back to bed and to sleep.

6

*Communication Between the Physician
and the Patient's Family: Introduction*

The seminar which I conducted for the sophomore medical class on "What a Cancer Patient Expects from a Physician" lasted for an hour-and-a-half. (My wife, by the way, participated as representative of a patient's family.)

At its conclusion, a student came up to me.

"Dr. Sanes," he remarked, "do you know that your entire seminar can be summarized in three words?"

"Three words?" I queried defensively.

"Yes," the student replied, "the three COM's—

"1. COMpetence,

"2. COMmunication,

"3. COMpassion."

The second of these three "COM" expectations, from the standpoint of communication, means communication between the physician and the family of the cancer patient as well as the patient himself.

For some physicians, communication with the family of the cancer patient is the most difficult expectation to meet—more difficult than communication with the patient.

In a letter dated May 6, 1976, to the editor of *The New York Times,* Mrs. Virginia Bekus of North Brunswick, N.J., wrote:

"I have been going to doctors a good part of my life, what with children, husband, parents, etc. I can say that although I have pressured for information, I received none; that although I have pressured for patient education or communication, I have received none. I have learned that doctors are a secretive group."

I do not know Mrs. Virginia Bekus. She gives no specific details of her medical experiences . . . whether cancer was one of the health problems in her family. She offers no factual evidence by which to judge the validity of her generalization that "doctors are a secretive group."

I do, however, know the wife whose 30-year-old husband died four months after diagnosis and onset of treatment of a testicular embryonal carcinoma with metastases, discussed in the previous chapter.

The physician who first saw her husband and worked him up clinically refused to communicate with her at all during the 12 days of his hospitalization prior to transfer by a consulting urologist to a cancer institute.

Ironically, the physician was a family practitioner who, in the past, had also seen the wife as a patient. He held a faculty appointment at a medical school in its department of family medicine.

The wife had no criticism of the scientific competence

of her husband's physician. Within a couple of days after promptly admitting his patient to the hospital he had carried out a diagnostic investigation, arrived at a clinical impression and called in a urologist for consultation and operation. He made daily pre- and postoperative visits to the patient.

But the wife has never ceased being critical and feeling bitter about the physician's failure to communicate with her. As a result of her experience, she shifted her own patient-doctor relationship to another primary-care physician.

A skeptical reader may characterize the foregoing illustration of physician-family communication as consisting merely of anecdotal evidence, involving only one patient, one physician, one family, obtained through a couple of informal interviews with the wife by a not-disinterested interrogator and reported by him as part of a personal narrative.

Let's look at some evidence which is more objective. It was reported by Shirley J. Salmon, Ph.D., at the 1975 meeting of the International Association of Laryngectomees, American Cancer Society. Dr. Salmon is speech pathologist at the Veterans Administration Hospital, Kansas City, Mo.

Her study of a group of cancer patients (largyngectomees) and their spouses in regard to physician communication grew out of an experience with one of her own patients.

He staggered into her office early one morning and, speaking with his artificial larynx, said ". . . you didn't tell me it was going to be like this. Why didn't you tell me?"

A short time later she heard similar poignant complaints from the spouses of laryngectomees attending a group workshop.

"Why," they asked repeatedly, "didn't somebody tell us how it would be?"

To determine how common such a feeling was, Dr. Salmon conducted a questionnaire survey.

Questionnaires were returned by 59 laryngectomees (10 of them women), from 18 states, and by 47 spouses (including 5 males), from 15 states. Eight of the laryngectomees were single. The average age of the laryngectomees was 60 years, of the spouses, 58 years. One-third of the married laryngectomees had two children at home at an average age of 13 years when the operation was performed.

I excerpt certain findings from Dr. Salmon's study of physician-patient-family communication.

More than 50 percent of patients said that their doctors discussed *only* the surgical procedure, while 36 percent said they were told that their operation could be life-saving, heard something about the "pathology" of their lesion and the prognosis. Just 49 percent of the spouses were given information by doctors about the operation, prognosis, and resumption of activities by the patient.

Fewer than one-third of the patients and fewer than 20 percent of the spouses received any additional information prior to surgery.

Of those who did receive information preoperatively, 30 percent of the patients and 13 percent of the spouses felt they were "well-prepared" for their experience. About 44 percent of the laryngectomees felt "poorly prepared," "not prepared at all" or refused to comment. Thirty-eight percent of the spouses felt "poorly prepared." An in-between group of laryngectomees and spouses felt "adequately prepared."

Sixteen of the 47 spouses, virtually one-third, indicated that they received no post-operative information.

There can be no question that some physicians, perhaps more than we in medical education and practice might want to admit, find it difficult to communicate—to talk frankly and sufficiently, and helpfully, with the family of a cancer patient.

Why is this so? Why is there this difficulty—even at times failure—in communication by physicians?

A number of factors singly or in combination may be responsible.

Let me suggest a few.

1. Even before applying for admission to medical school, some individuals, through inborn and acquired influences, develop a type of personality that will inhibit or prevent them from responding openly and confidently, understandingly and compassionately to patients and their families as total, intimately-related, interdependent human beings, especially in a chronic, serious illness like cancer. The decision to enter medical school doesn't change their personalities.

2. It is theorized that certain individuals actually decide to go into medicine because of their own fears of incurable illness and death. Feeling as they do, possibly

with their fears aggravated by what they learn and experience in medical school, they find it difficult or impossible to speak out on these subjects when they become physicians.

Tabitha M. Powledge, research associate at the Institute of Society, Ethics and Life Sciences, refers to one study that has shown physicians are "more afraid of death than other people," including "people who are terminally ill."

3. In medical school or teaching hospital, the average prospective practitioner learns little, if anything, from instructors and "attendings" through precept or example about the importance of communication. He gets few hints on how he can fulfill his responsibilities in this area when dealing with patients and their families.

What Dr. Jimmie Holland says in *Cancer Medicine* holds as true, maybe more so, for the family as it does for the patient.

"Conventional medical education has done little to equip the young doctor with knowledge of how to convey diagnosis of a potentially-fatal disease or how to offer continuing emotional support along with physical care."

A 1976 SUNY Buffalo Medical School graduate confirms this. At no time during his junior and senior years in didactic or clinical instruction was he exposed to information or practical examples in regard to communication with families.

If a resident learns anything about communication during his hospital training, he generally does so by himself. What he learns depends on his own attitudes toward the physician-patient-family relationship and his own trial-and-error experiences.

When I was a senior medical student about 50 years ago I worked as a clinical extern in a 900-bed municipal hospital. Residents were assigned to "lobby call." That meant being stationed in the hospital's main lobby during visiting hours to answer questions from patients' relatives. The assignment, though not a popular one, did at least bring residents face to face with families—acquaint them with questions and concerns of relatives including those directed to problems beyond the physical condition of the patient—and impress some with the definite need for communication. The assignment has long since been discontinued.

Individual physicians at a voluntary hospital often find transparent excuses for shifting the responsibility for talking to the patient with a grave disease and his family to their residents, who in turn pass it on to assistant residents, and so on down the ranks. The family may be left with a nurse or a medical student as the chief or sole source of information, advice, and support.

Recently I asked a surgical resident in a voluntary teaching hospital what he had learned from his "attendings" about communicating with the family of a cancer patient.

"Well," he replied with a cynical laugh, "I'll tell you. I've learned how, when I become an attending surgeon, to let my resident do the communicating."

4. Increasing specialization during the past 25-50 years along with advancing biomedical science and

technology has had a bearing on the problem of physician communication with all patients and their families, not alone those confronted with cancer.

In 1930-31 the Buffalo General Hospital, then, as now, a voluntary teaching hospital affiliated with the UB Medical School, filled only four residency programs: internal medicine, general surgery, gynecology, and pathology. All were of one year's duration and each took one resident. (There were also 12 rotating interns on the house staff.)

In 1976-77 the Buffalo General Hospital furnished residency training in 17 specialties and three subspecialties for the respective number of years prescribed by the various "Boards." It has 119 house officers of its own and circulates an extra 106 residents from other institutions through its programs. (The title "rotating intern" has been discarded in graduate medical education.)

Today in the U.S.A. there are 65 areas of certification for specialty in medicine.

General practice has become a specialty in the primary care area with internal medicine and pediatrics.

How much longer will we be able to accept many internists as primary care physicians? The American Board of Internal Medicine now offers certification in nine subspecialties. Often an internist so certified confines his whole practice to his particular sphere of interest. Will the general internist soon become an anachronism?

Two situations contribute to the bearing of specialization on communication.

Today, when a health problem arises, many persons go directly to a specialist. If their problem doesn't fall into his field, or if they need additional help, he refers them to another specialist, and so on.

Some primary-care physicians relinquish their relationship with a patient and his family after they refer the patient to a center, clinic, group or specialist. This is particularly true if the patient has a chronic serious disease like disseminated recurring progressive cancer which requires frequent outpatient visits, new and complex treatments, periodic checkups, multiple hospitalizations, and sophisticated diagnostic-laboratory procedures.

Social medicine blames increasing specialization along with advancing biomedical science and technology for causing "fragmentation, discontinuity and depersonalization" in the management of disease and the care of the sick human being and his family.

To the average practicing physician, these terms have become little more than cliches.

To the patient and his family, however, "fragmentation, discontinuity, and depersonalization" carry deep and distressful meanings.

These were well expressed by a fellow patient of mine, a bowling alley attendant in his mid-40s, husband and father, with stage IV progressive Hodgkin's Disease of three years' duration and severe familial diabetes mellitus of 22 years' duration.

"You gotta drag yourself from one doctor to another. . . . Some doctors you never see twice. . . . And what you get is mostly undevoted [*sic*] care."

I have deleted the interspersed profanities.

A specialist may see a patient only one or two times within the limits of his own area of scientific competence, sometimes only for one symptom or physical sign, one laboratory result, one diagnostic procedure, one type of therapy, one consultative opinion.

He may not even perceive the patient as an integral part of a family, may not be aware of a spouse, parents, children, brothers and sisters.

In the hospital he may call on a patient when the family is not present. If it is, an accompanying nurse may shoo them out into the corridor when the specialist enters the patient's room. In leaving he may pass by them without acknowledging their presence. He seldom if ever makes house calls to view the patient and family in their natural setting.

Increasing specialization along with advancing biomedical science and technology can therefore result in many patients and their families never having a physician to oversee and coordinate the various aspects of their medical situation, to act as a concerned, compassionate, continuing source of information and psychologic support.

Fortunate are the patient and family who do.

How much of a role specialization plays in today's medicine and how much physicians differ in communicating with a patient and his family is well illustrated in the following case history.

I interviewed the widow of a physician about one-and-a-half years after his death from carcinoma of the large bowel with metastases.

Her husband had lived two-and-a-half years after the onset of treatment. During that time the widow remembered 11 physicians who participated in the management of her husband's disease, from a general internist for the patient's original complaints through ten clinical and laboratory specialists and subspecialists, including a psychiatrist for the patient's suicidal moods in the terminal stage. There may have been several other specialists and subspecialists whom the widow never met or couldn't recall.

The widow gave a satisfactory grade in communication only to the general internist. He made himself available day or night to the patient and his wife from the first time he saw them in his office through the patient's multiple hospitalizations and between hospitalizations in the family's home to which he finally came to pronounce the patient dead.

She gave the lowest grade in communication to an internist who, because of his subspecialization in medical oncology, should have had the most empathy with cancer patients and their families.

He proffered practically no information and evaded all questions to which the patient and his wife sought answers—on recurrences, metastases, side effects of chemotherapy, prognosis. It was not until the wife became angry and demanded answers that he deigned to give them any information at all.

Before any reader jumps on me for some of my foregoing remarks on increasing specialization and its bearing on communication, I want to stress that as a physician-pathologist of 45 years I fully recognize—and as a cancer patient in remission with a three-and-a-half year survival I gratefully acknowledge—what progress specialization along with biomedical science and technology has brought in the past 25-50 years to prevention, detection, diagnosis, treatment, prognosis and rehabilitation.

The overall "five-year cure" rate for cancer has gone from one in five patients during the thirties to one in three since 1956.

For certain types of cancer—childhood leukemia, Wilms' tumor, osteogenic sarcoma, Hodgkin's Disease, non-Hodgkin's lymphoma, choriocarcinoma, carcinoma of the cervix—survival statistics have improved appreciably.

There has been substantial progress in other fields of medicine as well as advances in living and working conditions of people. Americans now enjoy the highest life expectancy and the lowest death rate in U.S. history.

I raise only one question.

Must the price for this scientific progress against disease be holistic, humane care for the patient and his family? (I know that being a specialist or subspecialist need not exclude one's being a complete physician. I always remember the late Dr. A. H. Aaron, internist-gastroenterologist, as an example.)

5a. Communication can be a special problem for a physician who has had a close personal and social relationship as well as a professional one with a patient and family for a long time.

This is particularly apt to happen when the physician is a general practitioner in a rural area or small town.

Such a physician may diagnose chronic myelogenous leukemia in a senior high school student whom he delivered, immunized against childhood diseases, and treated for colds, fevers, and broken bones.

Besides being for years the doctor of the patient's parents, he may serve on the local school board, hunt and fish with the father and know the mother through church and civic affairs.

Even in a metropolitan community such personal and social relationships may occur. A physician and his patient or a member of the patient's family may belong to the same town and country clubs. They may play golf or cards together, share the same hobby—antique automobiles, chamber music, firearms, miniature trains. They may meet and dine at each other's homes, go on joint vacations.

A registered nurse with disseminated lymphosarcoma (stage IV) wrote me about her experience.

"When my doctor, a friend, advised me with tears in his eyes of the diagnosis and prognosis ('three years to live'), he told me that he could not bear to tell George, my husband."

Because of the physician's inability to communicate, the wife had to do it herself.

5b. Communication often breaks down completely when the patient is a physician or member of a physician's family.

This may be partly because the attending or consulting physician is a friend of the physician-patient or of the physician whose relative has cancer.

It may be, though, that he simply assumes that all physicians, regardless of type of practice or of years out of medical school, know all there is to know about a specific cancer and that therefore there is no need to elaborate when they or a member of their families become ill.

But, really, how much ought anyone expect a psychiatrist, neo-perinatologist, bariatrician (et al.)—not necessarily a long time in practice—to know about the latest information on immunoblastic sarcoma with monoclonal gammopathy or, for that matter, adenocarcinoma of the rectum with which he or his wife is afflicted.

In the lymphoma-leukemia group to which my lesion belongs, most of present-day knowledge, and procedures related to pathologic classification, nomenclature, clinical diagnosis with closed and open staging, histologic grading, surgical-radiation-chemo- and immuno-therapy with side effects and complications, use of blood products, etc., didn't exist 5-25 years ago.

An otolaryngologist, out of medical school 40 years, made it a point when laid low by a life-threatening intestinal illness to caution his gastroenterologist:

"Forget that I'm a physician. I really don't know anything about my condition or its treatment. I may be a 'doctor' to you, but in looking after me . . . in talking to me and my wife . . . please think of me as a 'mister.'"

A physician who has cancer and members of his family can be just as vulnerable as lay persons to the mental, emotional, economic and other effects of the disease, sometimes more so. Lack of proper communication intensifies that vulnerability.

117

A Physician Faces Cancer in Himself

A physician in his 50s discovered a small node in his neck while shaving. A biopsy showed lymphosarcoma. Further workup indicated that the disease was disseminated.

The physician became too depressed to function. This, he decided, was it. He walked the floor at night. He worried about money. How much of what he had been able to save would his illness eat up? He had always had the notion that unless he provided well for his family financially, practically in perpetuity, he would fail them. He considered suicide, debated how much of the sedative that had been prescribed would be a lethal dose.

Most of his problem stemmed from the fact that he was a physician being treated by physicians who were also personal friends. They wouldn't or couldn't talk honestly to the patient and his wife about what they were doing and why, or about what lay ahead. No one was making any clear-cut, firm decisions, neither his doctors, his wife nor least of all himself.

If he refused to take the prescribed drugs and dosages, perhaps because of the side effects, the physicians (nurses too) acquiesced to his whims without explaining why the drugs were necessary, what they would do.

Finally his wife, in desperation, turned to a friend with disseminated lymphoma whose disease had been in remission for some time.

The patient-friend talked to the physician, told him that suicide was a poor solution, that lymphosarcoma need not be hopeless.

The physician accepted from his fellow patient the assurance his physicians had been unable to give him.

In time he learned to regard his disease more realistically. He followed the prescribed treatment. As his disease was brought under control, his depression disappeared. Two years later his disease was in remission and he had resumed full time practice.

6. Sometimes a physician's communication with patients and their families is affected by the arrogance which he adopts in his manner and behavior. This arrogance may spring from the healing and life-saving quality of the service he renders, professional and academic recognition and power, income and financial status, deference from his aides—nurses, technicians, secretaries, residents and students—social position, the reverential attitude of the public, etc. (May the seeds of arrogance be planted already in incoming first-year medical students when, at an orientation session, they are hailed by a faculty member as "the elite"?)

7. Lastly, some physicians may think or find themselves too busy professionally or personally to spend time communicating with patients and their families. They don't take the initiative themselves and if the patient or a family member does so they "didn't get the message" or "forgot to call back."

I'll describe two examples.

—A 34-year-old woman felt a small lump in the upper median quadrant of her breast and telephoned for an appointment with the family's primary care physician, an internist in group practice.

He saw her without delay, scheduling her at the end of office hours for examination of the breast.

The husband sat in the waiting room.

"I can't tell . . . it might be cancer," the internist, feeling the lump, told the patient. "You'll have to have a biopsy."

He wrote the name of a surgeon on a piece of paper, handed it to her, and walked out of the examining room. He passed the husband in the waiting room but seemingly didn't see or recognize him. He did not stop to speak.

The wife continued to sit silently in the examining room. She felt all choked up. ("A lump in the breast," someone has said, "is a lump in the throat for any woman.")

Finally the physician's receptionist came in. "Are you still here?" she remarked in surprise.

"Why, yes," the patient responded tremulously. "Isn't the doctor coming back to talk to me?"

"No," the receptionist said, "he has gone to keep a dental appointment."

The patient and her husband left the office. Instead of having the biopsy made by the surgeon recommended by their internist, they had it done by one whose name they obtained from a next-door neighbor at a hospital with which their internist was not associated. (The lump proved benign.)

—A middle-aged physician was hospitalized for biopsy of an enlarged axillary node. He went home after an overnight postoperative stay. In the afternoon of the next day, his doctor, a general internist, reported the

final pathologic diagnosis was lymphoblastic lymphosarcoma.

His wife, Jane, an executive in a business enterprise,
was at work. When she came home at 5:30 PM he gave
her the verdict. She panicked emotionally. She wanted
to know more. She was afraid that her husband wasn't
telling her the whole truth.

Picking up the telephone (the time was now 6:30
PM) the physician-patient dialed his internist at home.
The internist, besides being a professional colleague,
was a social friend of the couple, as was his wife.

The wife answered the telephone. The physician-
patient, addressing her by the first name, explained why
he was calling.

"Could Bill speak to Jane and clear things up for her
about the diagnosis?" he asked. "She's awfully on
edge."

"We have guests for dinner," the wife replied. "Bill is
busy mixing drinks for them. I'll give him the message.
He'll call back."

He never did.

Had he forgotten? Or had his wife failed to give him
the message?

On the following day the physician-patient, perhaps
somewhat pressured by his vexed wife, transferred himself to an internist (medical oncologist) for treatment
and care.

It was six months before he and his wife saw and
spoke to the original internist and his wife at a social
function.

There was no mention of the telephone call to the

internist on the night of the diagnosis. The couple still has no answer to their question. Why didn't he call back?

I must be fair.

Sometimes communication with the family of a cancer patient is not a problem which lies in the physician's personality, his attitudes toward illness and death, medical education and training, specialization, personal and social relationships with patient and family, arrogance, lack of time, handling of messages, etc.

Rather, it's a dilemma imposed upon the physician by the cancer patient himself who requests that the family not be informed of his disease.

What to do in such instances is the doctor's dilemma.

Here are two examples of how physicians handle it.

—Lilyan Tashman was a Ziegfeld Follies girl and Hollywood movie star. Upon learning that she had an inoperable, terminal cancer of the stomach, she wanted to keep the diagnosis from her husband, Edmund Lowe, stage and screen actor. The doctor, however, told Lowe the truth. The actor never let on to his wife that he knew.

—A general surgeon in his early 50s developed a chronic progressive degenerative disease of the central nervous system and was forced to give up practice. He and his wife moved from their home to a small apartment where she, a former nurse, took care of him. A married son lived in California, a daughter attended a New England college.

Two years later the wife noticed enlarged nodes in her neck and entered a hospital for diagnosis.

Left alone, her husband had to be admitted to a nursing home.

The wife's illness was diagnosed as disseminated lymphoma.

She remained in the hospital for X-radiation and the initiation of chemotherapy.

When friends brought her husband in once a week to visit her, she arranged her negligee to conceal the enlarged lymph nodes in her neck. He had no idea of the diagnosis and treatment of her illness. She asked her attending physician not to tell him.

The physician complied with her request. He did communicate fully, however, with the son and daughter.

After discharge from the hospital the wife gave up the apartment and joined her husband as a fellow patient in the nursing home.

Legally a cancer patient's request that his physician not disclose diagnostic and other information to family members comes under "privileged communication" and must be so honored. The physician, however, can try under ordinary circumstances to convince the patient that disclosure will redound to the benefit of the patient and to that of his family and doctor.

In the case of Lilyan Tashman, the physician took it upon himself to tell Edmund Lowe because, in the face of impending death, the actress had decided to go on a trip around the world with her husband for a second honeymoon. Aware of his wife's disease, Lowe could be ready for any contingency.

7

Communication Between the Physician and the Patient's Family: Why, When and Where?

My wife, who is a science writer, tells me that the first thing a student of journalism learns about communication is that it involves the answers to six questions—"the five Ws and an H: why, when, where, who, what and how."

If a newspaper reporter answers those six questions satisfactorily, my wife assures me that his readers will understand and empathize with what he has written.

Let's see if what works for a reporter communicating with the lay public is as effective for me, a physician communicating with other physicians about *their* communication with cancer patients and families.

Incidentally, only one student asked about communication with a cancer patient during the half-hour question-and-answer period that concluded my April, 1976 seminar for the sophomore medical class. Not one directed a question to my wife who participated as a representative of a patient's family.

Furthermore, in all my years in general teaching hospitals, there was never, so far as I can recall, a clinical conference on communication with cancer patients and families for attending physicians, house staff, junior and senior medical students. (Of course at my present age I can't rule out the deleterious effects of cerebral atherosclerosis on my recent and remote memory.)

I was particularly struck by the remarks of senior class representative Thomas Raab at the 131st Annual Commencement of the UB School of Medicine.

Conventional medical education, Raab said, has done little to prepare the young doctor for conveying a diagnosis of a potentially fatal disease or for offering continuing support along with medical care.

I assumed that Raab (now Dr. Raab) based his remarks on his own observations and experiences and those of his fellow students at our school in the past four years.

There could be no better witness than Dr. Raab—as medical student and graduate—to pass judgment on the teaching of communication, specifically with the cancer patient and family.

Dr. Raab is himself a patient in the same leukemia-lymphoma clinic I attend at the cancer institute. He has Hodgkin's Disease stage II in remission. The diagnosis was made in the first part of his junior year in medical school, November, 1975. He had a biopsy of a mediastinal mass (mediastinoscopy) staging laparotomy with splenectomy, supervoltage mantle X-radiation, oral and intravenous chemotherapy. Yet he completed his junior and senior years with satisfactory grades on time. And he was graduated with his class, which honored him by

choosing him its representative to speak at the commencement exercises.

I haven't had anything to do formally with undergrad-
uate medical education since my retirement from UB in
1971.

I've heard and read a lot about courses being introduced into today's medical curricula to teach students
communication with and compassion for patients with
chronic, serious, potentially fatal disease and their families.

These courses go by various names in various
schools—"personal and social medicine," "death and
dying," etc. (I'm not sure whether any are offered to
SUNY Buffalo medical students.)

I wonder, though, how many of the students who take
them feel that they have gained any real insight into
meeting the needs of future patients and their families or
whether they, as Dr. Raab remarked about his four years
of medical education, still feel unprepared at graduation.

While referring to physician-patient-family communication, I shall focus primarily on the physician's
communication with the family of a cancer patient.

As for my credentials—

It was not my professional responsibility as a pathologist to communicate the results of my cancer diagnoses
directly to patients and their families. Nevertheless I
sometimes did so.

Normally the pathologist communicates his findings,
opinions and advice to the patient's attending physician.

But not always. I can cite rare occasions involving
the pathologic diagnosis of cancer in fellow professionals or members of their families in which attending

physicians—often close friends—abdicated their responsibility and asked me to tell the patients or relatives the diagnosis.

More frequently, especially when the malignant lesions were unusual, attending physicians referred fellow professionals or relatives to me for consultation after telling them the diagnosis. Sometimes the professionals or relatives came without referral to talk things over.

Basically, communication with a fellow professional or his family in regard to cancer involves the same considerations as communication with a layman and his family.

In addition to my experience as a physician-pathologist, I have my experience as a cancer patient.

I have observed how physicians communicated with me and my wife and with other patients and their families, especially in the lymphoma-leukemia outpatient clinic where, for the past four years, I have been treated and checked regularly—on the average every two weeks.

My observations have been supplemented by what I have read since the diagnosis of my disease. This includes articles and books written by other patients and families as well as physicians, social workers, nurses, clergymen, et al.

Finally I can now look at the problem of communication from a third point of view.

I can look at it from the point of view of a member of the immediate family of a cancer patient.

A Physician Faces Cancer in Himself

In September, 1976, my only brother, 67 years old—the same age I was when my disseminated reticulum cell sarcoma (histiocytic lymphoma) was diagnosed—telephoned me at 7:45 AM about a genito-urinary complaint.

Within a half hour we were in the outpatient urology clinic of a local hospital. After a brief examination the attending urologist admitted my brother to the hospital for a medical workup. The diagnosis: leukemia. My brother was transferred to a cancer institute where his spleen was removed. He is now receiving chemotherapy similar to that which had been prescribed for me three-and-a-half years ago.

Today we are followed in the same lymphoma-leukemia service and outpatient clinic at Roswell Park Memorial Institute. Sometimes we are seen on the same morning. This can cause problems. Once, because of confusion over the same last name, the laboratory mixed up the reports on our blood counts, to the temporary consternation of our respective physicians.

So, if you will accept me as qualified, I'll proceed to answer the "five Ws and the H" of communication as I see them.

Of necessity there will be some overlapping of answers.

I don't mean to be all-inclusive, dogmatic or simplistic. What I have observed and experienced personally may not apply equally to every physician-patient-family situation.

Situations may vary, depending upon the individual

kinds of patients and their families and the types of cancer, treatment, course and prognosis.

Although my answers to the "five Ws and the H" are personal ones, perhaps not absolutely relevant to every patient or family, I do believe that they possess general validity and applicability.

Why?

The physician has not only a professional and moral responsibility but also a legal obligation (at least in New York State) to communicate the facts of cancer diagnosis, treatment and prognosis fully, comprehensibly and continuously to the patient and/or his family.

The legal obligation is stated clearly in Point 4 of the 15-point American Hospital Patient's Bill of Rights which, incorporated in the New York State Hospital Code, bears the force and effect of law.

Point 4 of the Bill of Rights reads "[that the policies and procedures at the hospital shall afford a patient the right] to obtain diagnosis, treatment, and prognosis in terms the patient can be reasonably expected to understand. *When it is not medically advisable to give such information to the patient, the information shall be made available to the appropriate person in his behalf.*" (The italics are mine.)

(Under ordinary circumstances the cancer patient has the legal right to decide what should be disclosed about his illness and to whom.)

If a physician, through oversight or deliberate lack of communication, should fail to fulfill Point 4 of the Patient's Bill of Rights in a state like New York, where it is considered as law—particularly if information is requested from him—the patient and/or family could under certain conditions have recourse to the courts.

Lay persons today, as medical consumers, are not only aware of their legal rights. Because of the mass media and public health education in schools, and through the American Cancer Society, health departments, medical societies et al, they may know more about cancer as a health problem, be more up-to-date in their knowledge, than some physicians.

When they or members of their families become ill, their questions can no longer be brushed off by patronizing, god-like statements from the physician: "Now don't you worry about anything" or "That's my business—you're paying me to handle that. I'm the doctor" or "I'll do the worrying . . . you just leave everything to me."

Communication should include not only the giving of the facts of the diagnosis and management of the disease but help in understanding the treatment, course and prognosis. It embraces continuing professional attention, information and referral for certain practical problems which may arise (transportation, financial assistance, etc.) and psychologic support and reassurance.

The patient who knows his diagnosis and understands his disease with its treatment and prognosis is better able to cope and adapt to it than the patient whose physician keeps him in the dark.

And the knowledgeable, understanding family is better equipped to give him the day-to-day care and support he needs. In so doing the family is at the same time helping to preserve and maintain its own well-being, stability, unity, perhaps its very existence.

The physician, too, benefits from free and open communication with the patient and the family. They will have more confidence in him, accept his recommendations and carry out his orders more faithfully. He may even get better diagnostic, therapeutic and prognostic results in the patient. Avoidance or lack of communication, on the other hand, may lead to feelings of uncertainty, helplessness, fear, anger and even alienation toward him. The patient, through his own choice or at the family's behest, may change doctors, hospitals, even go to a medical quack.

Let's take four examples of various approaches and results of physician-patient-family communication.

1. A professional woman of my acquaintance, in her mid-50s, underwent an operation for removal of a growth in her uterus. She was single, living alone, and the only surviving member of her immediate family was a brother.

Her physician, an attending surgeon in a voluntary teaching hospital affiliated with a medical school, never told the patient or her brother that the "growth" was a cancer and had already metastasized. (This was before the adoption of the Patient's Bill of Rights.) He led them to believe that he had removed a "tumor" and, because he didn't use the word "cancer," they assumed that the tumor was benign.

The patient failed to improve postoperatively. After her return to her apartment she felt herself growing weaker every day. Her surgeon told her that this was expected after an operation. She didn't believe him. This, she knew, was more than the usual postoperative lack of strength. If the surgeon couldn't recognize the difference, he obviously didn't know his business.

Urged by her brother she made inquiries about admission to an out-of-town nationally-known medical center, hoping that physicians there would be able to determine more accurately the nature of her illness and treat it more effectively.

She did not discuss her plans with her surgeon, but she did talk about them to a friend, also a professional woman, who worked in a field allied to medicine.

The friend, who suspected the true diagnosis, decided to intervene. She telephoned the physician, whom she knew through her work, and told him that he was about to lose a patient, and why.

He clearly resented her intrusion into the case, but upon thinking it over decided to talk frankly with the patient and her brother. He excused the fact that he had not done so before on the grounds that "they never asked me if the tumor was cancer."

After the initial shock of his announcement, the patient accepted the prognosis. Her belief in her physician was restored. She decided to stay with him. She accepted his explanations, followed his instructions and palliative treatment faithfully. (At the time hormonal- and chemotherapy were not available.)

Through her brother she made arrangements for daily care at home. She looked after personal, financial, legal and religious matters. She got in touch with relatives whom she hadn't seen for years or with whom she had even been at odds.

The disease worsened, but when her strength permitted she wrote notes of appreciation to friends who had stood by through her illness. In some instances she even wrapped little remembrances for them—possessions of hers that they had admired.

When death finally came, her brother delivered the notes and the packages.

"It was so much easier for both of us after we knew the truth," he told one of the recipients.

2. If communication is so important when the patient is terminal, how much more so it is when the patient has some hope of living, even if only a remote one but possibly for an extended time.

For example I know three patients with stage III-IV lymphoma (a nurse, a clergyman and an educator) who have gone 10-15 years on surgery, radiation, steroids and chemotherapy. All have been able to continue working in their respective fields. The side effects of treatment have often been discouraging, but their families have sustained them.

At the cancer institute one of my young fellow patients recently admitted to the lymphoma-leukemia clinic often becomes depressed because of the side effects of his experimental chemotherapy. At such times he tells his physicians that he is going to give up treatment, return to his home outside of Buffalo and die.

His wife, mother of their two children, has been fully informed from the beginning about his diagnosis and prognosis. She knows that the chemotherapy, though unpleasant, offers his only chance of survival. She won't let him give up.

He always returns to the clinic for further treatment. If he attains a 10-year-or-more survival, he will have his wife to thank.

3. Today, when my own disease has been under control for four years, my wife tells me that if she had not been fully informed of the nature of my illness and its treatment she might have been driven to leave me during the early days of my deepest depression.

She says that she would not have understood my retreat into myself, my lack of interest in her or in our life together. She would have felt that somehow she had failed me, was not making me happy.

4. The fourth example, a middle-aged registered nurse on the West Coast (one of the long-term survivors referred to earlier) has had lymphosarcoma stage III-IV for 12 years. She has been treated with surgery, radiation, steroids and chemotherapy.

On November 26, 1976, she was readmitted to the hospital for study and evaluation of chronic, intractable diarrhea and persistent fever.

"At that time," she wrote me two months later, "I

cared very little about what happened to me. It was as though my illness had a negative effect on what normally passes for rational thought."

The diarrhea was attributed to intestinal changes caused by radiation, the persistent fever to chronic bacteremia.

During the workup, a carcinoma of the rectosigmoid area was diagnosed.

"The surgeon was unwilling to do much with me until I was physically prepared," she continued, "and last but not least he wanted to make sure my attitude toward the surgery of the large bowel lesion was conducive to trying to get well, particularly since there was a 50% chance that an abdomino-perineal resection and colostomy would be needed.

"By December 9 the surgeon and I were both satisfied that I was ready and a six-and-a-half hour operation ensued. Fortunately the surgeon was able to do a sigmoid resection and end-to-end anastomosis without colostomy.

"Needless to say the hours I was in the operating room were a far greater ordeal for my family than for me. . . .

"By December 31 I was finally allowed to go home and at last I have moments when I can think clearly and even write a letter . . . I do feel better in general . . . Life again seems worth a try and I'm glad to be around.

"My husband had the most influence on changing my attitude, but several others were more than helpful. After all, my husband, too, needed support.

"Our son [the only child, in his 30s] came for a few days from the East Coast and was very important in this episode.

"A major source of help came from my sisters,

brothers and their spouses, all of whom remained with my husband and son during the entire six-and-a-half hour ordeal of surgery.

"Another influence was a few good friends. Their concern and support to my husband and myself extended not necessarily to visits but to keeping track of us, seeing that cooked food was available. They were always helpful and unobtrusive.

"The surgeon spent considerable time helping me to understand what he was trying to do and why. He leveled with me at all times and kept me abreast of all his plans for my care. He also took time to talk with my husband and kept an eye on his state of psychologic progress.

"I've been more than overwhelmed and grateful and wonder how more cancer patients can get this support from physicians, families and friends."

Let me briefly summarize what I have been saying, at the risk of being repetitious.

There are three, not two, parties involved in the diagnosis, treatment, course and prognosis of cancer.

They are the physician, the patient and the family (which I extend to include close friends, and fellow patients with their relatives).

All benefit from good communication.

The physician because the patient and family are more comfortable with him, more trusting and co-operative, willing and able to carry out his recommendations and orders and to recognize the limitations of today's medical science against the disease. The family member who assumes day-to-day care of the patient can be virtually a physician's associate and save him time, worry and effort.

The patient because he can look at his disease more objectively and more realistically, with less irrational fear. It is easier to face the known than the unknown. His physical as well as his mental and emotional well-being may be fostered by his own knowledge and understanding and by the care and support of his family.

The family because the chance of silences, suspiciousness, bitterness, estrangement between them and the patient and among themselves is reduced and because they have an essential part to play in the care and support of a loved one.

If the outcome is not a happy one they are better prepared in all ways—mentally, emotionally, economically, socially, legally, sexually, religiously and philosophically—to face the progressive course of the disease, the death of the patient and what lies ahead of them in life.

Here's one of the important things I've learned as a physician-patient.

On the average, cancer patients and their families complain more frequently and vehemently about lack of communication and compassion in a physician than about his scientific competence. And some of them seem never to forget that lack.

When?

The responsibility of communicating freely, comprehensibly, fully and compassionately with the family of a cancer patient (as with the patient himself) is not a one-time thing.

It begins with the patient's first visit and continues throughout his life and even beyond. The physician may, in the long run, spend as much time with the family as with the patient.

Here are some of the times when communication is particularly important.

1. At the time of the original workup.

The family should understand what the physician is looking for, the necessity and results of examinations and laboratory tests.

2. Before biopsy, exploratory surgery or treatment by surgery, radiation, hormones, immuno- or chemotherapy.

Dr. Shirley Salmon, whose study of the spouses of laryngectomized cancer patients was referred to earlier, found that their greatest interest was in having more information from the beginning. They wanted to know the surgical procedure, how the patient would be changed after surgery (anatomically, physiologically, psychologically and in appearance), what the problems of communicating and caring for him would be, whether he would be able to talk again and how to cope with personal and family problems that would arise postoperatively in the hospital and at home.

3. After biopsy or surgery.

The most difficult time for a spouse or other members of the family is the waiting period during and after surgery when they receive no information or emotional support.

I saw one family in the waiting room, anxious and

agitated, at 2 PM. They had come in at 7:30 AM, before the patient was taken to surgery. Six-and-a-half hours later no one had told them that the patient would be taken to the recovery room after the operation, and they could not understand why he had not returned to his room. No physician had come to talk to them and the busy nurses on the floor had little time or patience for their questions or perhaps had no information themselves.

4. As soon as possible after "cancer" is pathologically verified.

It is well to remember, however, that bad news is best borne in the daytime, when it is light, when people are around and there are things going on. Night with its darkness, silence and seemingly interminable length is a fearful time, especially if one is alone. Some of the fears are real, but many are phantom, irrational ones. If the family is given bad news in the daytime, they can seek aid and comfort from others and by night will be somewhat adapted to it.

If I were telling a family that a pathological report said "cancer," and I received that report at 5 PM, I'd wait until the next morning to break the news unless there were professional or personal reasons for urgency—e.g., the patient was to be transferred from a general hospital to a cancer center by ambulance in the morning.

It is important that pathologists get reports out as soon as possible. I wonder how many of them recognize what patients and families go through emotionally while waiting for a tissue report, even that on a suspected small basal cell cancer of the skin. Yet they are sometimes told casually that such a report will "take a week or so."

If there must be a delay, the family should be alerted to how long it may be and why. If other opinions are being sought in the locality or out of town, this should be explained.

5. In subsequent days when the shock of the verified pathologic diagnosis has diminished somewhat.

The family will want and need to know about additional types of treatment, either primary or adjunctive (e.g., radiation or chemotherapy), if these are needed, who will give them and where, what they will cost. The family should be informed, too, about how long the treatments will continue, what the side effects will be and the possible results.

6. Throughout the course of treatment.

The family should be kept in touch with the patient's response, any new developments or changes in treatment, prognosis or even in the personality of the patient.

7. Through follow-ups, even when the patient is not under treatment and the disease is "under control, in remission or cured."

8. When the patient is losing ground and starts to go down hill for any reason, either the disease itself or side effects and complications of treatment.

Ironically it is at this time, when the family most needs him, that the physician sometimes ceases to communicate entirely and gets out of the case.

9. During the end stage, when the patient is moribund or comatose.

It is important that the physician notify the family of

impending death as accurately as he can and do what he can to make things easier for them—perhaps extending special visiting privileges at the hospital so that they can be with the patient when they wish to be there.

10. At the time of imminent death.

The family should not feel that the physician has abandoned them, although there may be nothing further he can do scientifically to change the outcome.

A woman now in her 60s whose husband died 25 years ago has never forgotten that their personal physician, a family friend, didn't even come to the hospital during her husband's final hours.

Notified at his home of the imminent death, he told the resident to make the patient as comfortable as possible, that there was nothing further he could do. *He* hung up the phone. Although the wife of the patient was standing at the nurses' station while the resident was speaking, the physician didn't inquire for her. She was crestfallen and bitter.

An older physician who knew the couple socially but had not been involved in the care of the patient stopped by while making rounds. Sizing up the situation, he stayed with the wife for a while, giving her the support she so needed.

11. Even after death.

The family may need to be reassured that everything possible was done for their loved one and that they themselves performed well, providing not only the needed care, but encouragement, support and love.

This final communication may also mean a great deal to the physician, Dr. Morris A. Wessel says:

"The physician who so often feels defeated by medicine's failure when a patient dies may find positive satisfaction in continuing his relationship with and supporting the remaining members of the family as they grieve, mourn and regain equilibrium. Bereaved family members . . . appreciate knowing that their doctors care about them and wish to help them at this difficult moment.''

Finally, a practical matter.

The family that gives permission for an autopsy is entitled to receive the results or a summary of them in terms they can understand.

Often their request that they be informed of the findings is overlooked. The resident who obtained the consent may forget to mention it to the pathologist or attending physician.

A young widow whom I interviewed for this article told me that when she failed to receive the report of the autopsy on her husband which she had requested she mentioned it to her family doctor. He had not been on the team that treated her husband, but he asked for and received a summary of the autopsy findings, copies of the summary sheets in the protocol, which he gave to the widow. He didn't explain them, and she hesitated to ask what they meant, but simply put the summary with her other papers. When she told me about it, and showed me the autopsy protocol's summary sheets, I gave her the first explanation she had.

Such explanations come best from the physician who treated the patient, not from the pathologist. A good time is a couple of weeks after death when the autopsy protocol is usually completed with gross, microscopic and other findings. The spouse or other family member should be encouraged to ask questions.

Where?

The "where" of physician-family communication will vary with the "when."

Such communication may take place in the physician's office, general hospital, cancer center, extended care facility, nursing home, hospice or family residence.

It may even, when the family cannot be physically present, take place over the telephone, by telegram or cablegram or through the mail.

In the case of the 85-year-old man with cancer of the colon referred to earlier, the surgeon at the university hospital never met the patient's wife, physician-son or two daughters. He communicated with the wife and son by telephone and mail and they communicated similarly with the two daughters, one of whom was out of the country.

In the four years since my diagnosis, my wife and I have spent the months of December, January and February in Guadalajara, Mexico. During those months, our communication with my physician at the cancer institute has been solely by mail.

When I leave home I take with me his office and home addresses and telephone numbers. He has mine in Guadalajara as well as those of my Mexican physician.

So far we have not had to resort to the telephone, but

every two weeks I send him, by air mail, a report on my physical, X-ray and laboratory findings. If he wants further information or wishes to suggest further diagnostic procedures or treatment, he contacts me, as he did this past year. My wife is fully informed of the contents of all our communications.

When a fellow patient at the institute, a college student, was found to have leukemia while in school in the Midwest, his physician there telephoned his parents in Buffalo to discuss the diagnosis and outlook with them.

The parents of another college student were on a "round the world" trip when a diagnosis of malignant melanoma was made on him. The physician's cable reached them in Italy.

If physician-family communication is to take place in a public facility, as it often does, the area selected should offer privacy, quiet and comfort.

The wife of the 30-year-old patient with testicular embryonal carcinoma cited previously was grateful for the promptness, frankness and sensitivity of the urologist at the cancer institute in communicating with her and her husband on his admission.

She said later, however, when I interviewed her, that it would have been easier for them both if the discussion could have taken place somewhere besides the solarium-dining room on the urologic floor.

It is difficult to listen, to ask questions and assimilate answers, to experience and express emotions about a serious, potentially fatal diagnosis in such a setting.

Other patients and their visitors are chatting, having lunch, coming and going. The television set is turned on, possibly to a soap opera or jocose game show.

It is even worse to get serious news, as many families do, in a hospital corridor, from a surgeon still in operating room garb making rounds—or in a hospital lobby from a physician "on the run," entering or leaving the hospital.

Some hospitals and cancer centers realize this. They set aside areas where physicians can talk, privately and quietly, with patients and families.

The lymphoma-leukemia clinic that I attend has such a room, tastefully and comfortably furnished, like a doctor's office, completely separate from the main waiting, examining, treatment and physicians' conference rooms.

Good physician-family communication doesn't always require such a formal setting. During follow-up visits of outpatients, the physician at the institute may call the family member, sometimes at the request of the patient, into the examining or treatment room to discuss how things are going and what is being done.

When a patient is hospitalized, his room, if it affords privacy, may be the setting for communication.

But some patients may elect to remain in their own homes. This poses more of a problem.

Today's medical students and young physicians look upon house calls as a thing of the past, of no value to the physician, patient or family.

House calls, however, are still indicated for certain

types of patients. One of these is the advanced, bedridden cancer patient.

Dr. J. Englebert Dunphy, past president of the American College of Surgeons, believes that such visits should be made at regular intervals by the family physician and from time to time, if possible, by the surgeon or oncologist who undertook the definitive care.

"The value of a visit to the home of the patient on the part of the surgeon," he says, "is unbelievable. . . . I can testify that the reward to family, patient, referring physician and surgeon is one that cannot be put into words."

8

Communication between the Physician and the Patient's Family: Who?

Who?

In answering the question "Who?" we must consider both the giver and receiver of information and support.

The first is the physician—or those members of today's medical team whom he calls in for communicating in their special fields of expertise.

The second is the family member or members who deserve, seek and need information and support.

If the family of an adult patient has a primary-care physician (family practitioner or internist), I feel that it is his responsibility to provide or arrange for the principal communication with the family from the first complaint throughout the course of the disease.

Even when specialists enter the picture, the primary-care physician should retain his relationship with the family, visiting the patient daily when he is in the hospital and continuing his visits, as needed, after the patient returns home.

Unfortunately many families today, in all socioeconomic groups, have no primary-care physician.

In such instances, the responsibility for the initial communication becomes that of the specialist who make the diagnosis and carries out the indicated treatment. Usually this will be a surgeon or a gynecologist. (The latter may act as a primary-care physician for his cancer patients and their families.)

When the specialist has communicated his findings, results of treatment, recommendations for further therapy and follow-up examination, estimate of the outlook as he sees it, etc., he may suggest that the patient and family find a primary-care physician (a family practitioner or internist-medical oncologist) to provide continuing and overall care. If the patient and family have no preference, he may make a referral or suggest that they call the County Medical Society for a list of names.

In either instance, the specialist should go over the pertinent aspects of the patient and family situation with the new physician—in person, in writing or by telephone. (If the patient already has a primary-care physician who referred him to the specialist, the latter should, of course, keep him fully informed at all times.)

But the fact that there is a primary-care physician doesn't free the specialist of all future responsibility for communicating with the patient and family. He should make it clear to them that he will continue to be available for follow-up examinations or consultations on problems in his field and that he will personally confer with the primary-care physician if referrals to other specialists are needed.

When diagnosis, treatment and follow-up are given in a cancer institute, medical center, university or government hospital—whether in outpatient clinic or inpatient service—communication may come chiefly from residents or fellows. Attending physicians—full-time or part-time—should, however, be available and accessible to the patient and the family. If there is a primary-care physician, he should always receive a full typed report promptly and should feel free to phone or come in to discuss the patient's condition.

In today's medical practice a physician does not have to do all of the communicating with patients and their families himself.

There are others who can be helpful to certain patients and their families—perhaps more helpful than he can be, either because they are more readily available and accessible or have special knowledge and skills in patient-family education, counseling, service, psychologic and spiritual support.

Among them are nurses (practitioners, educators, home visitors), admission and discharge co-ordinators, social workers, dietitians, clergymen, counselors (psychiatric, family), rehabilitation, prosthetic and vocational specialists, representatives of the American Cancer Society, patients, patients' relatives, et al.

By using them wisely the physician can save his own time and effort and serve the patient and family better.

The development and expansion of the "medical team" in recent years to include such ancillary members is a response to the patient's—and family's—need for the services they have to offer, services not furnished by many physicians.

Yet some physicians look upon such ancillary personnel as interfering in the physician's domain. They resent their efforts to help. This is true even in large general hospitals or cancer centers which have organized departments or staffs in ancillary fields.

One such oncologist heads a cancer service where some patients and families get little or no information, either in the hospital or upon discharge, about problems that lie ahead and how to cope with them. Yet when ancillary personnel, recognizing these needs, volunteer their services as communicators, the oncologist tells them:

"That's my business, not yours. I'll tell the patient and family what I want to tell them when I want to tell them and how I want to tell them."

Even physicians who regularly turn to ancillary personnel when a patient or family is medically indigent or on welfare may not think of involving them in the care of private patients and their families.

On the other hand, there are some physicians who may see the existence of such personnel as an excuse to abrogate their own continuing responsibilities for communication.

How do patients and their families feel about communication with ancillary personnel?

They welcome it if they need and want information and support that their physicians cannot or will not give them.

When being asked whom they would most like to have seen preoperatively, in addition to the physician, the largest number of 59 patients who had undergone laryngectomies for cancer and of 47 spouses voted for "another laryngectomee and spouse." Others whom they listed were esophageal speaker, speech pathologist, minister, counselor, artificial larynx speaker, New Voice Club member, American Cancer Society representative.

Ancillary personnel can smooth the path almost every step of the way. In the section on "When?" I didn't stress communication on discharge from the hospital, but later I overheard a conversation that indicated that here, too, ancillary personnel can play a very important role.

Some patients go home with little more communication from their surgeon than "You can go home now—I'm through with you."

Even this may come to them indirectly when a nurse enters and says, "The doctor has signed your discharge. You can go any time." The family may not even be present.

In contrast to this, the discharge co-ordinator on the head and neck service of the cancer institute whom I overheard covered everything, answered all of the questions a 70-year-old man and his son wanted to know. It was a perfect job. I was as moved by its perfection as I might have been by a Cezanne still life or a Chopin Nocturne played by Rubinstein.

Communication with ancillary personnel will not, of course, satisfy patients and families when it comes to information about the medical aspects and problems of their disease.

Here they want to talk to the physician personally. And the ancillary personnel with whom I have discussed the subject agree.

Such personnel do not view themselves as entering a patient-family stituation on their own, as replacing the physician.

They consider themselves members of a medical team

of which the physician remains the captain. They wish to be called in by him, to report to him, to consult with him, to be supervised by him, to have him answer the medical questions.

They want to help—but they want and expect the physician always to remain in the picture.

How long this co-operative attitude will continue I'm not sure on the basis of the hostility I hear expressed, especially by nurses, against physicians who do not communicate well or fail to seek assistance in communicating with patients and families. When a physician fails to come up to their expectations of a complete man—not just in scientific competence but also in his attitude and behavior as a person, in his communication and compassion—they are disillusioned and bitter. Certain leaders of the nursing profession are already speaking of the nurse as an autonomous professional.

(In fairness I must add that I interviewed the director and departmental heads of a metropolitan Visiting Nursing Association which offers comprehensive services. They told me that there are certain physicians who consistently initiate relations with and utilize services of the association for cancer patients and their families in the most effective ways and with the highest co-operation.)

The question of who in the patient's family should be the recipient of information is often answered by the patient himself, not always wisely.

He may, of course, refuse permission for any such communication.

If he does not, the obvious choice should be the person or persons who are closest in relationship and/or will be taking responsibility for the patient's continuing care and support. For most patients—but not all—that means the closest of kin—spouse, parents, son or daughter, brother or sister.

It may, however, be a more distant relative—a nephew or niece—or a close friend.

In these days of free life styles, it may be a "friend" who is living with the patient as a spouse, what we would once have referred to as a "common-law wife or husband."

In the case of a fellow patient of mine in the lymphoma-leukemia clinic of the cancer institute, a bachelor physician in his 70s, it could have been a housekeeper of many years (until his death not long after diagnosis.) She brought him to the clinic by automobile for his periodic checkups, waited to drive him home, looked after him there, visited him when he was an inpatient.

There will be times when problems arise and difficult decisions have to be made that the communicating family member will want to bring in others in the family.

I know of a daughter caring for a 90-year-old father who called in all of her brothers and sisters from various parts of the country, including one who was a retired physician, to help decide about a proposed treatment. The father was too confused and upset by the diagnosis to make the decision himself, and she didn't want to accept the responsibility on her own.

In another instance, a wife and mother, facing the

imminent death of her husband, asked the physician to talk to their two teen-aged sons.

The physician himself, sensing a special need, may suggest that he talk to the family as a whole.

Not all family members are able to cope. In some instances the physician may recognize at the onset or during the course of the disease that the responsible family member or members selected as recipients of his communication and as providers of care and support cannot face the knowledge of the facts and the practical problems involved. They may even want out of their responsibilities, though they hesitate to say so.

This is not strange. Even certain physicians and nurses can't face looking after advanced-terminal cancer patients professionally, let alone those nearest and dearest.

But it's more than a matter of mental and emotional adaptability. Age, physical strength, general health, background and experience, training and skills, available time and other factors may also play roles.

The wife of an elderly patient, for example, may find it well-nigh impossible to get him from bed to a wheelchair, to handle a colostomy, to give hypodermic injections or even to read a thermometer.

When this becomes obvious, the physician should explore with the patient and involved family member or members, the social worker or visiting nurse, whether there is anyone else who might take over some or all of the care functions. Thereafter the communication about these functions would be between the physician and whoever is selected.

The patient's failure to ask the physician to talk to

the family or the family's failure to ask questions shouldn't be taken by the physician as an easy way out of an unpleasant, unwelcome duty.

He has a legal, professional and moral responsibility to communicate with the family unless specifically requested not to do so.

I believe that this is true even when the patient is a physician himself. A patient, whether a lay person or physician, should not be expected to do all his own communicating with the family. Nor should a member of the family be left to tell the patient the diagnosis or to communicate other crucial information about the course and progress of the disease.

One final word.

If the patient is a close relative of a physician who is not involved medically, it is only professional courtesy, if the patient has no objection, to keep that physician informed of the diagnosis and course of the disease. This can be through face-to-face conversation, telephone, or, if the physician lives at a distance, by letter.

In my own case, perhaps because I am a physician with some know-how in the field, perhaps because of the personalities involved, communication at the cancer institute has generally been excellent.

My physicians have told me what I needed and wanted to know. There has been no need to rely on ancillary personnel for specific information, although they have been continually helpful in encouragement and support.

My wife has shared fully in the communication. (I have taken it upon myself to keep my brother and sister informed.)

Although my wife does not accompany me on my regular clinic visits, she has been present at every decision-making stage to hear what was being discussed, ask questions and contribute her own thoughts.

She went with me on my first visit to the institute for history and physical examination. The next week, after closed staging, my medical oncologist and therapeutic radiologist told us, together, what they proposed to do, why and the results to be expected.

Later, when I developed, in succession, shingles with rising fever, a type of Lhermitte's syndrome, acute abdominal pain (bowel obstruction) and a critical level of pancytopenia, she as well as I participated in discussions of what was to be done.

Before my recent splenectomy, my regular clinic oncologist, the head of the service, and the surgeon who was to operate met us jointly and told us what they planned to do and why, answered all of our questions.

During my hospitalization they communicated their findings twice daily. At least one of those times my wife was present. When a urologic problem arose, my medical oncologist called my private urologist to discuss it with him.

On the morning of my discharge, my surgeon, who was on his way out of town, came into my room and told me everything I wanted or needed to know. He discussed how things looked, what to expect, restrictions on activity. He wrote out a prescription and made an appointment, precise as to day and hour, for my post-surgical checkup—an appointment that the floor nurse confirmed in writing before I left. When I had to excuse myself to go to the bathroom because of "antibiotic diarrhea," the surgeon stayed on to answer my remaining questions through the closed door.

On my checkup visit at the clinic a week later, the surgeon and my medical oncologist together talked frankly with my wife and me, answered our questions, assured us that we could call either of them at any hour of the day or night if we were worried or if anything untoward occurred.

9

Communication between the Physician and the Patient's Family: What?

What?

At all times the physician should tell the responsible family member or members the truth as far as it is known.

That means during the initial workup, at diagnosis and throughout the entire course of the illness.

My wife has always wanted such communication. Indeed, she has insisted upon it, not only from my physicians but also from me as a physician-patient. She has also kept abreast of developments in the field of lymphoma by reading medical textbooks and journals and talking to other patients with the disease.

It is true that my wife's background and knowledge are different from those of the average family member of a cancer patient. She is the wife of a physician and has been a medical reporter for 36 years.

But what she wants in communication is what the responsible family members of most cancer patients want. This is true even if they cannot bring themselves to question the physician because they feel in awe of him or think he is too busy to be bothered, or because they are in a state of psychologic shock or depression.

Last week a former neighbor, the wife of a public high school teacher who had been a high school teacher herself before the birth of her three children, telephoned my wife and me. (She knew that I had cancer.)

Her 75-year-old mother, an alert, active widow living alone on the other side of the city, had consulted a rheumatologist about pain in the back and ribs. He admitted her to the hospital for diagnostic tests, then told the daughter—but not the mother—that he had discovered "cancer of the bone with anemia."

The daughter was so overcome that she couldn't collect her wits enough to ask for further explanation. The rheumatologist immediately referred the mother to a medical oncologist in a group practice on the staff of another hospital.

From the daughter on the phone came all of the questions she had failed to ask the rheumatologist and had had no chance, as yet, to ask the medical oncologist.

What kind of bone cancer was it—the specific type? How long did her mother have to live? What quality of life could she expect? Would there be pain? Could she continue to live alone in her house? How would the disease be treated—chemotherapy—transfusion? What side effects and complications might the mother suffer? How much would the treatment cost? What were the advantages and disadvantages of treatment by a private physician and in a cancer center? How long and how often would the mother have to be in the hospital? Should she be told of the diagnosis and outlook? . . . .

159

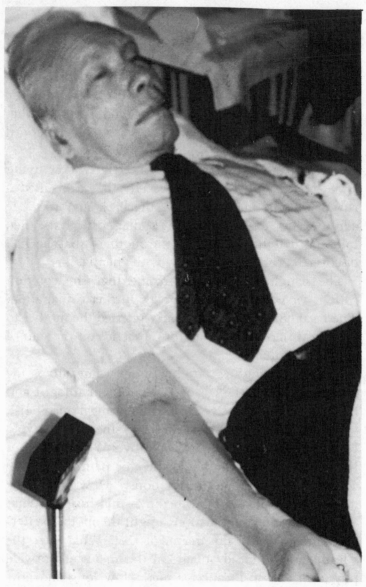

On July 27, 1977, as an outpatient, Dr. Sanes received his first transfusion of two units of packed red blood cells (note the needle in the vein of the right forearm).

"Wait a minute," we told her. "Make a list of all of your questions. Ask your mother's present physician, the oncologist, to answer them to the best of his knowledge. Telephone his office. Maybe he'll answer the questions over the phone. If he's busy, perhaps he'll call you back. Or his secretary will make an appointment for him to see you in his office or at the hospital."

In a few days the daughter telephoned us again. Her mother's disease, she said, had been diagnosed as "multiple myeloma."

"I did as you advised," she said. "I made my list and called the physician's office. He was busy, but he called me back. He answered my questions frankly and honestly on the phone—except that he was unable to make any estimate of what the drugs for chemotherapy might cost. He will tell my mother the diagnosis so that she can participate intelligently in all decision-making."

In some patients it is not only desirable but imperative that family members be given all of the answers.

This was true of the 90-year-old father referred to previously who was too confused and upset to understand the diagnosis of metastatic cancer of the neck, source undetermined, and the options open to him.

Even with a young, seemingly well-adjusted cancer patient, capable of understanding and making personal decisions at the time of diagnosis, and along the course of illness, a situation may arise which requires the physician to communicate with a family member.

This was true of a 40-year-old wife and mother who suddenly developed a visual defect in one eye after she had been under treatment for lymphoma for some time.

She drove with her husband the 50 miles to the cancer

161

institute. It was not the day of her regular appointment and they had to wait while someone located her physician. She sat silently beside her husband. Neither spoke. When the physician arrived, the visibly distraught wife went into the examining room with him.

"What did the doctor say?" her husband asked when she reappeared.

"He said that the eye . . . Oh, I don't know what he said . . . Why didn't you come into the room when he examined me?" she wailed.

In his relationship with a family member or members, a physician ought not be just a scientific diagnostician and therapist. He should also be an all-around compassionate communicator. He should supply factual information, educate, advise, counsel, make arrangements and referrals, support the family psychologically.

He should never forget that the etymological derivation of the word "doctor" is from the Latin word meaning "teacher."

The doctor should be prepared to answer the questions the family asks (no question is unimportant to them) and also the ones it does not ask.

His answers will help the family care for and support the patient, anticipate problems and cope with them, look after and preserve its own well-being and integrity.

Here is a list of "what" questions. (You will note that it includes most of those asked by the daughter of the mother with multiple myeloma.) Not all will come up during the course of every physician-patient-family relationship. Those that do come up may come up at different times. The list doesn't include all possible questions. I have implied, raised or answered others in previous articles and will do so in the next article on the "how" of physician-patient-family communication.

1. What examinations and laboratory tests will be done during the initial workup? Why?

If the diagnosis turns out to be "cancer," the family has been prepared to some extent. The psychologic shock will not be so great.

2. What is the diagnosis?

I believe that the family should be told the specific name and character of the cancer in terms that it can understand. It should know, for example, that it is dealing with "multiple myeloma," not simply "bone cancer." Family members often gain considerable satisfaction from "researching" what has been written about the disease in Merck's Manual, the public or medical school library, NCI-ACS pamphlets or from one of the public information services set up by NCI-ACS or a cancer center. If they have been given too broad a diagnostic category they may be confused and even angered by discrepancies between what they have been told by the physician and what they have learned elsewhere.

3. What are the options regarding consultation and management of the disease? What other physicians and institutions might be considered?

While the final decision rests with the patient, if he is

163

capable of making it, the family often has considerable input in arriving at that decision.

4. What, if anything, is known about the cause of the disease?

If industrial or agricultural factors are or may be involved, the answer to this question may be important to the family financially and in terms of its own health.

The family of an asbestos worker with carcinoma of the lung, mesothelioma or GI cancer may be entitled to financial redress. And because asbestos particles are known to cling to workers' clothes when they leave the plant, persons exposed to those particles in the home may want to undergo physical examination themselves.

If there is a possibility that a genetic or familial factor plays a part in the cause and development of the disease, others in the family should be alerted. This is true of close relatives of a patient with cancer of the colon due to heredo-familial polyposis, or the daughter or sister of a patient with carcinoma of the breast.

I often wonder about the possible etiologic or pathogenetic factor(s) in the reticulum cell sarcoma (histiocytic lymphoma) and the hairy-cell leukemia (leukemic reticulo-endotheliosis) diagnosed in myself and my brother respectively when we were the same age.

If the cause of a specific type of cancer is not known or proved, it is equally important to communicate this to the family of the patient.

A husband may be worried that his fondling of his wife's breasts in love play caused her mammary cancer. The wife of a 65-year-old patient with carcinoma of the colon who reads somewhere in the recent popular press of high fiber cereals being touted as preventives for such cancers may blame herself for not having fed her husband any bran during their 40-year marriage.

These seem like silly examples, but I have run into both of them, and even sillier ones.

Fearful of being confirmed in their guilt feeling, family members may hesitate to ask the question that is troubling them. The physician should recognize their anxiety, determine the cause and answer the unasked question.

5. What does the physician propose as primary and adjunctive treatment for the cancer—surgery, radiation, chemo-, hormonal, immunotherapy, a combination of these, or experimental therapy? What about reconstructive and rehabilitative, supportive and palliative treatment?

The family should understand that the management of cancer, even the same type of cancer, may differ in different patients.

6. What are the possible frequent, temporary or permanent, tolerable or serious side effects, complications or sequelae of the proposed type of treatment?

In some instances these factors may cause more problems than the disease itself.

Patients undergoing radiation therapy, chemotherapy or both may experience side effects ranging from nausea, alopecia and fatigue to infections, pancytopenia or hemorrhages. During chemotherapy there is the danger of incompatabilities between drugs prescribed for the cancer and those which the patient may buy over the counter or another physician may prescribe for another condition.

Think also of patients undergoing surgical procedures such as mastectomy, radical head and neck or gynecologic operations or abdominal-perineal resection with colostomy.

The colorectal service at a cancer institute has a check list of items to be carried out before performing abdominal-perineal resections with colostomy.

One of these is to talk with the family.

A sequela for the male, they indicate, may be impotence.

Even such a relatively trivial thing as a stitch abscess can be alarming to the patient and family who have not been told that it may occur. (There's nothing "trivial" to an uninformed cancer patient and his family.)

An elderly man living in a small town underwent a laparotomy at a cancer center about 250 miles away. One night—several weeks after he returned home—he noticed as he was getting ready for bed that his undershirt was stained red and yellow. The stain overlay the inferior end of his healed incision at the umbilicus where he couldn't see clearly. So he asked his wife to look at it. She saw an opening in the incision through which blood and pus oozed and a couple of "black things" that she couldn't identify.

Instead of waiting for morning to see the local family practitioner or to telephone the surgeon at the cancer center, she got her husband up in the middle of the night and hustled him off by automobile to the cancer center where a surgical resident without ado cleaned up the perforated abscess, removed two loose black sutures and sent the couple home with the assurance that all was well.

The oncologist who treated the 75-year-old widow with multiple myeloma referred to earlier could have spared her and her daughter much concern and agitation if he had warned them that there can be side effects to a supportive treatment such as a blood transfusion.

The patient had a transfusion in a teaching hospital affiliated with a medical school, then went home. Within a short time she felt feverish and developed chills which made her shake. She called her married daughter in considerable alarm, not knowing what was happening to her. She didn't associate the symptoms with the transfusion but with her disease.

The daughter, leaving her children, drove over posthaste. When she saw her mother shaking, she telephoned me.

I asked if her mother had a fever. She said that her forehead felt hot, but there was no thermometer in the house.

I told her that her mother was probably having a transfusion reaction. (I could speak from personal experience. I had had such a reaction myself.)

I suggested that she call her mother's oncologist and check.

She phoned me back and told me that she had called the office of the group with which the oncologist practiced and been informed that since it was Thursday, he had the day off and wasn't available. Meanwhile she had gone out and bought a thermometer and taken her mother's temperature. It was 101° orally, and she was still having chills.

I told her that the oncologist must have someone taking his calls on his day off and suggested that she call the group again.

In a short time she was on the line to me. She had telephoned the group and found that the oncologist did have a regular back-up physician, in fact, an associate, but he was unavailable because it was a religious holiday for him. This time the daughter explained her problem and the receptionist said that she would get in touch with another physician in the group who could prescribe Benadryl. In several hours the mother's temperature came down and she was soon feeling herself again.

7. What will management and treatment cost, in the beginning and throughout the course of the disease?

To my knowledge few physicians have any clear idea of the actual cost of the drugs and tests they order. A medical student, himself a victim of lymphoma, confirmed this for me by routinely asking the interns and residents with whom he worked the cost, to the patient or a third-party payer, of the treatments they prescribed or the operations in which they participated. None had any idea. Some were openly irritated at being questioned.

I can cite a personal example of the value of having an idea beforehand of the cost of a drug. My physician at the cancer institute prescribed a five-day course of

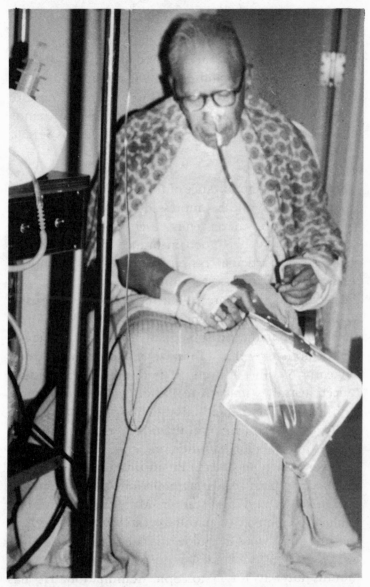

In the immediate postoperative period after his splenectomy, Dr. Sanes' chief complication was paralytic ileus. He retained a nasogastric tube for 9 days, had intravenous fluid for 11 days, a Foley catheter for 15.

Carbenicillin, explaining that the drug was "rather expensive." The information saved shock and the embarrassment of mind and purse that might have otherwise occurred when my wife went to a cut-rate drugstore to pick up the drug and found that even with my senior citizen's discount the cost of the prescription was $41.50.

8. What is the importance of follow-up examinations?

The family should be impressed with the fact that the threat of cancer never ends, even with a supposed "cure," and that it is good insurance to have periodic checkups. A particular cancer, supposedly in complete remission, may recur, even after five years. Some, like those of the colon or breast, may be multiple, appearing at successive times, or clinically mestastasize late. There are indications that in some patients radiation therapy or chemotherapy for cancer may, years later, cause leukemia or other cancers. It is for these reasons that cancer institutes make a real effort to keep in contact with patients and their families long after they have undergone treatment, encouraging them to return at regular intervals for examination.

A woman whom I met at the institute didn't look as if she had ever been sick a day in her life. But she told me:

"I'm like you. I have cancer. Mine is in the urinary bladder [non-invasive papillary carcinoma grade I]. I feel fine and I wouldn't know that I had cancer from the way I feel. But I come to my urologist every three months anyway for cystoscopic examination. He has impressed me and my husband with the need to keep an eye on things."

Patients with unexpected complaints following surgery and those on radiation-chemotherapy predisposing them to infections, etc. should be encouraged to make emergency telephone calls and visits if problems arise, without waiting for their regular follow-up visits.

9. What changes and limitations will the patient's disease and treatment impose upon his appearance, personality, physical functioning, working at his occupation or profession, school and university attendance, daily habits of living, diet, exercise, sports, sex, travel, social activities, interaction with family members and others? What can family members do in the face of these changes and limitations?

For just one extreme example, think of what it means to a patient who has undergone radical head and neck surgery, and to his family, to be hospitalized 300 miles from his home for several months while undergoing reconstruction and rehabilitation.

10. What problems may arise in the family as a result of the patient's disease and treatment? I have mentioned them before, but let me repeat. They may be physical, mental, emotional, sexual, social, legal, economic, religious, philosophic, etc.

In Dr. Shirley Salmon's study of laryngectomees (cancer patients), spouses were asked to indicate, in order of descending importance, problems for themselves and their mates which they saw to be a direct result of laryngectomy.

171

(Remember that the overall five-year survival-"cure" rate for cancer of the intrinsic larynx runs 70-85%.)

The spouses ranked speech communication the first problem, followed by social, psychological, employment, alcohol, sexual and financial problems. There was no indication that any of these problems would have existed if it had not been for the cancer and laryngectomy.

11. What source can the patient and family turn to for advice and help with such problems, in the medical care system or in the community?

The physician should be familiar with persons and agencies outside his own area of expertise or professional interest and should make that information available to the patient or family if or as the need arises. A printed form or brochure that lists addresses, phone numbers and persons to contact in the area can be most helpful. Roswell Park Memorial Institute and the State Health Department have prepared such a brochure for western New York.

The list includes State and County Departments of Health and Social Service, the Visiting Nurse Association, the County Unit of the American Cancer Society, the Leukemia Society, the State Rehabilitation Department, New Voice Club, Reach for Recovery and Ostomy groups, other cancer patients and their relatives, a number of voluntary community, family service and religious organizations, the Red Cross, Salvation Army, labor unions, private companies, et al.

For a number of years I served as chairman of the

Committee on Services to Patients in my county unit of
the American Cancer Society. All requests for service
were referred to me for a personal check with the patients'
physicians before they were granted. Nearly all requests
came from family members, on their own or through
non-medical persons. Only a few (actually I can't
remember more than two or three) were prompted by
the patient's physician.

12. What about the prognosis?

The physician's relationship with the patient and the
family throughout the course of the disease may depend
to a large extent upon how he answers this question. (In
any disease most physicians are primarily interested in
diagnosis and treatment. Patients and families are
chiefly concerned with prognosis.)

A physician must tell the truth derived from scientific
evidence and clinical experience. At no time should he
destroy hope by projecting personal feelings, fears and
hangups. He should not make unjustified predictions
based on his own lack of up-to-date knowledge and
experience in oncology.

Many physicians are altogether pessimistic and defeatist about cancer even before the lesion is thoroughly
evaluated from an oncologic standpoint.

You can see this when a physician is confronted with
cancer in a family member.

I can cite two instances from personal experience.

In the early years of the use of the "Pap" smear and
the concept of preinvasive uterine cancer, I reported to a

young physician that his wife had squamous cell carcinoma-in-situ of the cervix (previous class III smears). The physician, who worked in a highly specialized field far removed from gynecologic oncology, threw up his hands in despair. Yet this cancer approaches a five-year cure rate of 100%. Today the American Cancer Society omits carcinoma-in-situ of the cervix from its statistics of incidence and death.

Years ago a middle-aged urologist broke down in tears when he came to the laboratory to check a report of focal intra-epithelial carcinoma with slight superficial invasion noted accidentally in one microscopic section of the gall bladder which had been removed from his wife for chronic cholecystitis and cholelithiasis.

The wife was not informed of the cancer. There was no further treatment.

At that time the overall survival rate for carcinoma of the gall bladder was two %. But for focal superficial carcinoma with micro-invasion the survival rate was at least 50%.

The wife outlived her husband by years. He died unexpectedly from an acute hypertensive cerebral hemorrhage.

The two physicians mentioned above heard only the words "carcinoma" and "cancer." They reacted emotionally to the pathology of semantics rather than responding rationally to the semantics of pathology-oncology. To them "carcinoma" or "cancer" had the too-often popular connotation of an always progressive fatal disease with a short course. They failed to recognize that each carcinoma-cancer is a particular disease process in a particular patient in a particular medical setting with its own particular course and outcome.

There are many measurable variables which can and should be considered in arriving at a possible prognosis—duration of symptoms and signs, manner of detection or diagnosis, location (organ, site in organ, region), rate of growth, size, gross appearance, histo-cytopathologic type and grade, stage, kind of border microscopically, local and general effects—anatomical and functional, available methods of treatment, response to treatment, side effects, complications and sequelae of treatment, age and sex of patient, patient's physical and physiologic state—immunity, pregnancy, pre- or post-menopause, etc.

Further, in considering prognosis, the physician must also remember the still unidentified variables which we may classify under the term "luck."

On the day of my four-year survival from disseminated reticulum cell sarcoma I teased my clinic oncologist, "What do you think—the result of your scientific treatment or of luck?" A patient himself, with a nine-year history of Hodgkin's Disease, he replied smilingly, "Let's not exclude luck."

Metastatic cancer cells may lie dormant for prolonged periods. A certain percentage of cancer patients who refuse treatment survive five years. The medical literature contains reports of "spontaneous cures" of pathologically verified cancers.

Some physicians go so far as to translate their pessimism and defeatism into specific chronologic terms, perhaps in response to the exasperating demands of the patient and family for a categorical answer.

If such a prediction doesn't come true, the cancer patient and his family may make cynical and derisive jokes or vent anger and resentment about the physician's "dead in three years" or "six months to live" verdict.

(In his 1977 novel, *Madder Music*, Peter De Vries has a satirical passage in which his healthy "hero," imagining himself dying and wondering how long he has to live ponders the time-honored six-months-to-a-year.)

Hopelessness and helplessness may disorganize family life. They can send patients and families to other physicians or even lead them to consult quacks or to use scientifically unproven methods at a time when cancers may still be in controllable form.

Let me cite the experience of a fellow patient at the cancer institute—a 47-year-old man.

A surgeon in his home town in a neighboring state did an exploratory laparotomy on him and found a hepatoma. The condition was inoperable, he told the patient and his wife, advising him to "quit work, stay home and be comfortable as long as you can" since "you'll be dead in six months."

The patient had been in seeming good health. It just didn't seem possible. He was the head of a household of six persons. What would they do without him?

He and his wife were desperate. They considered Laetrile but finally decided, instead, to seek a second opinion at Roswell Park Memorial Institute.

"What can they do for you there?" his surgeon chided him. "They'll just experiment on you."

The surgeons at the institute were less gloomy. They removed the hepatoma with the left lobe of the liver. There was no additional treatment. Only follow-up visits were scheduled. The patient returned to his home and job. He engaged in his favorite sports of fishing, target shooting and motorcycling.

When, three years later, he complained of upper abdominal pain, he underwent a second laparotomy at the institute during which metastases were noted. He was placed on experimental chemotherapy. To date—five months after laparotomy—he continues a fairly active home and sports life. He has given up his job but he periodically drops into his previous place of employment to help out. Every month he comes with his wife the 300 miles from his home to the cancer institute. He takes his turn in driving the automobile. In Buffalo he and his wife telephone or visit my wife and me at our home.

A physician may feel that a given cancer patient may not live more than a short time after diagnosis. He has a right to express his opinion. But actually he is sticking his neck far out if he thinks that he can make an absolute chronologic prediction at the initial diagnosis and onset of treatment of what an individual patient will do with an individual cancer.

Dr. Roger Terry, professor of pathology, USC Medical Center, puts it aphoristically:

"Each patient is unique and each cancer that may develop is also unique."

False optimism in prognosis may be accepted more

tolerantly by patient and family than rank pessimism and defeatism, but the physician who is falsely optimistic may lose credibility, especially if the patient or a member of his family is knowledgeable about medicine—a doctor or nurse, for example.

Within the limits of available oncologic knowledge and practice, the physician, after considering the measurable and unidentified variables, can only predict statistically, on the basis of percentages and averages. He can only give odds. The individual cancer patient may surprise him. There have been inaccuracies in prognosis even in patients referred to hospices for end-stage care.

Here are two points in regard to prognosis which I picked up as a physician-patient in the adult leukemia-lymphoma clinic. (They would not have come to my attention in clinics for carcinoma of the lung, esophagus or pancreas, with constant overall five-year survival rates through the years of 5-10%, less than five% and one% respectively. Most patients with these cancers die within six months to two years of diagnosis.)

1. Prognosis for cancer patients may change for the better with the passage of time—even over a relatively short period, e.g. 5-30 years. There has been a definite change in the overall five-year survival rates of chronic forms of leukemia from the 1940s to the 1970s. For men the rate has risen from 14% to 30%, for women from 17% to 34%. In Hodgkin's Disease, during the same years, the overall five-year survival rate for both men and women has risen from 25% to 54%. In estimating prognosis for cancer, physicians must keep in mind the possibility of future progress against the disease.

2. Control in the management of a cancer at a certain time in the history of oncology is a more realistic goal than cure. This point can be emphasized in stating the prognosis for patients with leukemia and lymphoma and will contribute to their understanding and composure and to that of their families. A long-term fellow lymphoma patient expressed it better than I when he said to a husband waiting for his wife—a newly-admitted patient—to return from the examining room: "Maybe they won't cure you here . . . but they'll keep you living as long as possible."

So let's summarize the answer to our final question, "What about prognosis?"

Tell the truth as far as it is known from a scientific-clinical basis. Beware of personal, emotional influences which project pessimism and defeatism or false optimism. Preserve hope if possible. Take all measurable and still unidentified variables into consideration. Avoid specific chronologic predictions. Keep in mind the possibility of future progress in diagnosis and treatment. Set up control as a more realistic goal than cure at a certain limit of oncologic knowledge and practice. Never forget you're dealing with an individual cancer and caring for an individual patient and his family.

Now let's see how the foregoing points were reflected in the prognosis of my own cancer.

In February 1973, on my first visit to Roswell Park Memorial Institute, I asked the oncologist who examined me about the outlook for a patient with disseminated reticulum cell sarcoma (of the diffuse histologic type).

He described his informal prognostic classification of the lymphomas as "good" and "bad." Disseminated histologically-diffuse reticulum cell sarcoma (histiocytic lymphoma), he said, was not just a "bad" one; it was "the worst." He couldn't give me an absolute prognosis, but he would check the institute's computer for the most up-to-date percentages of survival with the latest therapy.

The next time I saw him he had the percentages of survival for one, two and five years. He didn't know whether he ought to disclose them to me. The overall five-year survival rate on the basis of the institute's experience, he said, was five %. Reports in the literature, however, were appearing with more hopeful results—five-year survival rates up to 10%. (My wife shared this information.)

I have now gone five years with my disseminated-diffuse reticulum cell sarcoma. It is in remission as far as can be determined medically. (There is no guarantee against relapse.)

Living, especially in the past year, has not always been easy, comfortable, happy or desirable. But until recently I remained fairly active and productive. From 1973-1977 my wife and I spent three months during each winter in Guadalajara, Mexico. I have never missed a *Buffalo Physician* press deadline for one of my articles.

I am sure that some of my physician friends, when they first learned of my diagnosis, gave me "six months to one year to live." I could read the prognosis in their faces and in their manner to me. Actually, in 1973 the computer's percentage for my six month to one year survival was 50%.

At the end of my second year of survival I ran into a physician on the street who hadn't seen me since my initial diagnosis. He greeted me in wide-eyed amazement, blurting out, "Gee, . . . you look great for a guy who is supposed to be half dead!" I didn't bristle at his remark. In fact, it cheered me. Originally the computer had estimated that in two years I would be three-quarters dead. It had prognosticated a 25% two-year survival rate.

The patient with reticulum cell sarcoma (histiocytic lymphoma) first diagnosed in 1978—only five years after the diagnosis of my disease—can hope for an altogether different prognosis from the one I received in 1973.

The contrast is made in the opening paragraph of a May 30, 1977, article in the JAMA. The first sentence abstracts an article in *Cancer* 30: 31-88 1972: "The (histologically) diffuse histiocytic lymphoma is the most virulent histologic form of lymphoma and few patients achieve remission with single-agent chemotherapy." The second sentence abstracts three articles published in 1974-1975 (*Lancet* 1:248-250; *Blood* 43:181-189; *Cancer* 35:1050): "It has recently been shown that patients with diffuse histiocytic lymphoma (even in advanced stage) who achieve complete biopsy-proven remission (with combination chemotherapy) often sustain prolonged disease-free survivals and perhaps cure."

The American Cancer Society in its 1978 "Facts and Figures" under "Treatment Trends" lists histiocytic lymphoma (reticulum cell sarcoma) among eleven tumors that formerly were considered incurable but that now are frequently controlled.

10

Communication Between the Physician and the Patient's Family: How?

How?

In answering the six questions involved in physician-patient-family communication—"the five Ws and the H"—it is the "H" that is most important.

The "five Ws"—the why, when, where, who and what discussed in previous articles—all lead up to the "H"—how to communicate. The "H" wraps up all the other elements of communication in one effective package.

The way we tell the patient and the family is as important as what, why, when and where we tell them.

"It isn't what he says that's the problem," one of President Carter's aides told a newspaper reporter earlier this year. "The problem is in the way he says it."

What is true for the President is just as true for the physician who wants to establish good communication with the patient and his family.

I am sure that you have deduced from reading my previous articles that as a matter of principle I believe in telling the whole truth in complete honesty. And for telling not only the whole truth but the same truth to both patient and family.

My wife and I both want to know the same truth. My physicians understand this. She tells me what she learns. I tell her what I think. We keep nothing from each other.

Not all physicians, and not all family members, believe that this is a good idea.

But even when such an attitude prevails, it is my observation from the experience of my wife and me and that of others I have seen in the lymphoma-leukemia clinic that I attend, patients and families are better able to cope when there is free and open, equally-shared communication.

The chief of that clinic has a hard and fast rule that he will not accept patients unless both patient and family know the diagnosis.

Sometimes either the patient or the family object to the other being informed.

When a college student was referred by a private physician who had not told him that he had leukemia, the parents, who knew, asked that their son be kept in the dark.

"It's so cruel to tell him that he has a fatal disease," the parents begged. "Please don't."

"I must," the chief of the clinic told them firmly. "Otherwise I cannot accept him as a patient."

The parents gave in, but asked that the physician inform their son privately. They could not bear to be present. He refused.

"I want to talk to the three of you together," he told them.

He took the patient and his parents into the small room in the clinic that is set up for just such purposes.

"You've been pretty sick for some time," he told the student. "Do you know what you have?"

"Leukemia," the boy responded calmly, without hesitation. Though no one had spelled his illness out for him he had known all the time.

Getting everything out in the open made things easier for both the patient and his parents. They could talk to each other again without trying to hide what they knew or suspected. Treatment continued in a regular manner. As Roman Catholics—the son was particularly devout— they gained psychological and spiritual comfort from arranging for a priest to visit the patient regularly— something they would have hesitated to do when they were trying to hide the truth from each other.

What I know or believe about the "how" of communication can be summed up in four maxims that I have learned from a journalist (my wife), a television producer, and two general authors.

1. My wife, with 38 years of experience as a communicator, expecially in writing about health problems, says that "the more and better the communication, the more and better information for making decisions."

2. When I first served as co-ordinator of a television program, *Modern Medicine,* the producer, a specialist in medical broadcasts for the public, told me: "Never underestimate the intelligence of your audience but never overestimate its information."

3-4. The two general authors wrote so as to qualify what some might find too harsh in my principle of the communication of the whole truth honestly.

The first said: "Honesty doesn't mean cruelty when it's truth with emotional support."

The second stated: "Painful truths should be delivered in the softest terms, and expressed no farther than is necessary to produce their due effect."

It is with these four maxims in mind that I have formulated my own credo as to "how" to communicate with cancer patients and their families.

If I were a public relations man preparing a television program to dramatize perfect physician-patient-family communication, I should probably start with an archetypal physician like Marcus Welby.

He would have a certain physique, beard and hair style, type of dress, voice, manner, knowledge and expertise in oncology, emotional stability, integrity, sensitivity, attentiveness to the individual and concern for the needs of others.

Undoubtedly there are such physicians in real life. I myself have been fortunate enough to find some who come close to such an ideal.

But I have to admit that most physicians do not fall into this perfect pattern.

Despite often superior academic records in school, scientific and technical success in postgraduate education and practice, many lack the ability to relate personally to patients and their families. Perhaps in some cases this trait has been taken out of them by an education that stressed science and technology over humanistic medicine.

Since we don't live in a world of idealized television programs, we have to work with what we have.

Doctors and patients and families are all human beings and all different.

The doctor who meets the needs of one patient and one family, professionally and in communication, may have no rapport at all with another.

I've seen this repeatedly during my five years of weekly or biweekly attendance at the lymphoma-leukemia clinic of the cancer institute.

Most of the average 30 patients and their families who come to the clinic daily are happy with the regularly scheduled physicians. Some, however, are satisfied only with a specific doctor. If he is absent they see another only reluctantly or refuse to be examined or treated at all.

I can cite two such cases, both patients in wheelchairs who had come a considerable distance to keep their appointments.

The first, an elderly woman, agreed to see another physician when the receptionist informed her that the physician she considered "hers" had been called away on an emergency. But after she had seen the designated doctor she sat in her wheelchair waiting to be picked up muttering, "I came all that way and then couldn't see my doctor—a fine thing!"

The second, a younger man, obviously very ill, adamantly refused to accept a substitute when informed that his regular physician was out of town.

"But all of our doctors are equally good," the receptionist told him.

"I don't care about that," he rejoined, "if I have a choice I want to see my own doctor, and if I can't see him I'm going home. I'll come back tomorrow when he's here."

The doctor the patient or family member insists on seeing may be the one that another refuses to see.

It isn't easy to meet the communicative needs of hundreds of patients with different problems and personalities, backgrounds and outlooks. This is particularly true when the doctor is dealing with persons facing and coping with a chronic, incapacitating, potentially fatal disease like cancer.

But if a physician can't be all things to all people, there are steps that he can follow to communicate more effectively with all of his patients.

Here are some of them.

Establish rapport.

During the workup, the oncologist or specialist should establish a personal relationship with the patient and family. One of the advantages of having a primary-care physician is that this rapport is already assured.

Be available and be on time.

The family shouldn't have to run around the hospital looking for the physician. He should make an appointment to talk to them and then, if possible, not keep them waiting unnecessarily.

A medical oncologist kept a newspaper editor waiting nearly two hours after the appointed time when he came in to talk about his sister's disease.

"I had cancelled some of my own appointments to go to the physician's office," the brother told me. "There was no one else in the waiting room. The physician was alone in his inner office and he remained alone. I heard him talking a couple of times on the telephone. The secretary informed him of my arrival and reminded him later, but he just didn't seem to realize that my time was valuable too."

Take time.

This is especially important when first explaining the diagnosis, course and prognosis.

Sit down with the family member. An elderly physician once told me, when I was a lot younger myself, "One minute sitting down is worth five standing up when speaking to a patient or a member of his family."

This is as true when making rounds as it is in your office.

Go through the formalities of introduction. Be calm and poised, open but not casual, objective but not cold, warm and concerned.

"Communion is vital in all true communication." A

consoling hand on the arm or shoulder of the person to whom you are talking can mean more than words in helping him accept what you are saying. Your TQ (touch quotient) may be more important than your IQ (intelligence quotient).

"He was all right, I guess, in giving information, but he was such a cold fish," a physician's widow said of the manner in which an oncologist who treated her husband during his terminal cancer communicated with her.

One physician, acting on the advice of his clergyman father, started out in practice by greeting his patients and their family members with a warm handclasp when he saw them in his office or in the hospital. Now, he says, they often reach out to grasp his hand before he has extended it fully.

Such gestures are particularly important in a university or governmental hospital or a cancer center where the patient may be assigned to a physician he has never seen or heard of. The physician will seem warmer and more concerned if he introduces himself by name, position and relationship to the patient or family member.

Avoid interruptions.

Your rapport with a cancer patient or a member of his family can be seriously damaged or utterly destroyed if you take too many "times out," even for professional purposes. And certainly they are not there to listen to a telephone conversation with your stock broker or a friend who wants to make a golf date.

Be truthful and honest within the limits of available knowledge.

The family may press the physician for definite answers on treatment, course and prognosis. Their own future plans depend upon what happens to the patient. The physician should tell them honestly, when he cannot give guarantees, that medicine is not an exact science but remind them that research is constantly going on.

Use simple, understandable English, not medical terminology or jargon.

The medical term may be more precise, more part of the physician's speech, but it may mean little to the patient or the family. Don't talk as if you were delivering a paper on the subject at an international meeting of your professional society.

This is true for even well-educated, otherwise sophisticated persons.

My wife tells me of a general news reporter with a considerable reputation in other fields who filled in for her on the medical beat one day, covering a seminar on cancer.

When he returned to the office to write the story, she asked him how things had gone.

"Fine," he responded. "The seminar was interesting and I learned a lot. But they kept using one word I didn't understand."

The word was "carcinoma."

A UB student majoring in psychology asked to interview me on tape about my illness. The interview was to be his term project for a class on "Death and Dying."

To his first question, about my diagnosis, I replied "histiocytic lymphoma."

He stopped the tape.

"Lymphoma," he asked, "is that cancer?" (Incidentally, he received an "A" on his project.)

Avoid expressing your thoughts and emotions in nonverbal forms which may upset the patient or family.

Watch your facial expression, tone of voice, even bodily movements. "One's face ofttimes says more than one's tongue." And in speaking to a wife or mother, do not take a patronizing, male chauvinistic attitude.

Incidentally, from my personal experience and observation of other patients, I have the impression that women physicians are more empathic than most men.

I remember one physician in his 40s with fatal cancer who derived most of his comfort, encouragement and support from the woman physician on the service where he was being treated. Perhaps he adopted her as a mother.

If the patient has cancer, say the word. And specify the type of cancer.

Don't evade or equivocate by saying "tumor" or even "malignancy." If you use a term like "lymphoma," explain that it is a type of cancer.

A husband and wife interviewed on national televi-

sion said that they went for months after being informed of the husband's diagnosis ignorant of the fact
that he had cancer.

"We thought it was only lymphoma," the wife said.

Unless the physician is very plain-spoken, the family
member may not grasp what he is saying, may shut out
of his mind what he doesn't want to believe. He may
accept "tumor" or "lymphoma" as something other
than cancer.

But when you do give a verdict of cancer, explain it.
All cancers are not equally life-threatening, and the
patient and family should know that. Correct any
misconceptions they may have.

A young wife I know was thrown into hysteria when
her physician told her that the small spot on her cheek
was "basal cell cancer" and didn't explain anything
more.

*Use a printed sheet or diagram to help get the
message across.*

The family and the patient himself may get more
from an objective, illustrated statement about the type
of cancer, stage, treatment, course and prognosis than
from what the physician tells them face-to-face. They can
read the statement at their leisure, when they are
calmer—re-read it if necessary.

Dr. Shirley Salmon's study indicated that pre- and
postoperative information needs to be presented in
writing as well as in conversation.

This is also true of directions for therapy. The

physician is not only the source of information but the source of instruction.

When I returned from the cancer institute in March I was taking a total of ten drugs, some as many as four times a day. In my mental and physical state I was unable to keep them all straight. It was up to my wife to administer them.

Some patients who aren't able to cope with the numbers and kinds of drugs prescribed have to be admitted to a hospital for treatment that might otherwise have been given at home. Repeated errors of administration when dealing with today's powerful drugs could be life-threatening.

Many clinics, including Roswell Park Memorial Institute, prepare pamphlets for distribution to patients telling them everything possible about their type of cancer, including after care.

Listen to the questions the family member asks and then answer them to the best of your ability.

Communication is aural as well as oral. It is important to listen as well as to talk in communicating with the family.

No question is unimportant to the family member asking it.

Answer as succinctly and briefly as possible, mentioning—but not dwelling upon—every qualification and reservation (except where more emphasis is required legally).

"Whenever I ask a doctor a straight-out question,"

one of my fellow lymphoma patients commented, "he takes 20 minutes to answer 'maybe.'"

Some family members, even some patients, will write out their questions ahead of time.

They may fear that, in the awesome presence of the physician, they will forget something that they want to ask. Or that the physician, busy and impatient, just won't wait for them to finish asking their questions orally.

If a patient or family member comes to you with such a list, don't put him down as a neurotic. Save his list and those of others who question you in this way, and write a book of answers.

It might be a best seller.

See that the family gets information, education, advice and counsel about non-medical problems that may arise as a result of the patient's cancer.

That means that the physician himself must be familiar with hospital and community facilities and able to communicate the facts about them to the patient and the family.

It would be most helpful if this could be done in written form, complete with addresses and phone numbers.

Give the family your telephone number.

Assure them that they should feel free to call if the patient's condition changes, if there are unanticipated side effects to treatment—infection with fever, hemorrhage or other medical problems.

A physician, particularly a medical oncologist, may want to set aside a "telephone hour" in the day during which he can take calls of a non-emergency nature without interrupting his regular office hours.

The lymphoma-leukemia clinic that I attend encourages patients and their families to phone their physicians when they have questions about their condition, particularly when there is any change in it.

I have done so myself on several occasions.

When I developed shingles after radiation therapy, my fever continued to rise for several days. At that point I called the clinic and was given a special appointment in the afternoon to avoid infecting others during morning clinic hours.

Another time I had a cold that hung on for several days with pharyngitis and laryngitis. Fearing tracheobronchitis, again in the face of a rising fever, I called my clinic physician at home at 7:30 AM.

Assure the family that you will stick with the patient and with them for the duration of the illness and beyond, as emphasized in the section on "What?"

Don't try to give all of the information at once. Be prepared to repeat at future times some of the information given during the first interview and to expand upon it.

The shock of learning the diagnosis may be all that the family can truly absorb at one time, even though they indicate that they want to know "everything."

Keep the family informed as to new developments, including changes in treatment and reasons for them.

Keep your promises to the patient and the family.

If you promise a report on the outcome of a biopsy, blood test or X-ray study at a given time, don't keep the patient waiting or forget about it entirely. He and his family will be on tenterhooks until they hear, even if you told them that you wouldn't telephone unless there was something abnormal. Call them anyway, as soon as you know the results.

Don't get angry if asked about a new proved or unproved treatment or procedure reported in the press or elsewhere and whether it could be applicable to the patient's case.

The family is constantly reaching out for any hope that it can find. It has no way of judging newly-reported knowledge other than asking about it. If the physician has information, opinion or judgment on which to reply to their question, he should do so. If not, he should tell them that he will look into it.

Don't get angry if a friend of the family intervenes.

This may happen when the patient and the family are passive persons who hesitate to trouble the physician because he is too busy or because of the awe in which they hold him.

I'm not a very assertive patient myself. I don't like to

complain. (I also fear being a neurotic.) Most often it is my wife who insists, when I have a problem, that I get in touch with the physician about it. When I have refused, or neglected to do so, she has sometimes gone to the physician behind my back. Without her, or a friend who would fulfill a similar function, often I would do nothing, perhaps brood and get worse.

My physician in the lymphoma-leukemia clinic recognizes this. He recently told me not to withhold my complaints or kid about them, but to tell him about whatever was troubling me.

Preserve hope, encouragement and support as far as possible.

No matter how well a physician communicates, he must be prepared for a variety of reactions on the part of the patient and the family.

Rarely, because of a family member's lack of knowledge and insight, he may not be able to communicate at all.

Novelist Peter De Vries writes in *The Blood of The Lamb* of the father of a leukemic child who met a 300-pound woman in the hospital lounge. She was pacing back and forth in a rumpled house dress, a cigarette with an inch of ash hanging from her mouth.

"Boy, dis place," she said. "When me and my little girl come in here she didn't have nothing but leukemia.

Now she's got 'ammonia.'" While the father listened unbelievingly she continued:

"Ammonia, dat's serious. She's in an oxygen tent and I can't smoke there. It's a tough break for her because like I say at first she didn't have nuttin' but a touch of leukemia. I don't believe I ever heard of dat before. What is it?"

For the patient and family who are capable of understanding, good communication will soften the blow, but it cannot assure the physician that they will always accept the news as he would have them accept it.

Here are some of the reactions he can expect from families.

No apparent reaction or denial. Some persons don't show distress at all. This may be because of their own inhibitions, their wish not to "bother the doctor," or their inward denial of what he is saying.

Psychologic shock. A wife's legs may collapse under her if she is standing when she learns that her husband has cancer. She may leave the hospital and go out in a snowstorm without her coat and boots. A man learning of a similar diagnosis in his wife may forget where he parked his car or be unable to drive it home when he finds it.

The husband of a registered nurse was "numb for three days" after learning that she had lymphoma.

When possible, it may be well to suggest that another member of the family or a friend who will be under better emotional control accompany the spouse to the interview.

Tears. Even strong men may weep upon learning that a wife or child has cancer. A medical student told me that when he went to his father's place of business to tell him of his diagnosis of Hodgkin's Disease "my father broke down and cried."

Anger or rage. The anger is against fate, but initially the physician may bear the brunt of it. He may be accused of delayed diagnosis, misdiagnosis, even malpractice. He may even be threatened physically. Be patient. The rage will abate.

Insistence on more communication, a second or third opinion, referral to another physician or to a medical or cancer center, a written report.

Don't respond angrily. Wouldn't you want to be sure if you received a diagnosis of cancer in a member of your family?

An obsessive desire to know everything that is going to happen, and exactly how and when.

A physician's wife with such an obsession made herself so disliked by the nursing and medical staff that eventually the floor nurses refused to have her husband admitted as a patient to their floor. They took her unsatisfied curiosity as obnoxious testiness.

I have focused on physician-patient-family communication at the initial diagnosis of cancer, the onset of treatment and throughout a relatively satisfactory course.

I have avoided the "how" of communicating with the family of the patient facing impending or imminent death.

I could have discussed this from personal experience. As a patient, I took a turn for the worse on February 19

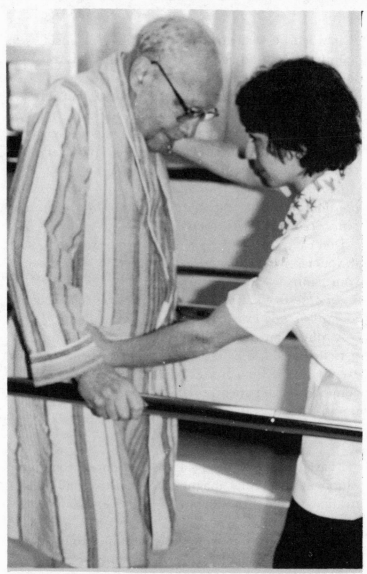

Dr. Sanes gained added reassurance, in the months before his death, from physical therapy. Here Susan Barr, director of the institute's Physiotherapy Department, helps him strengthen his muscles by walking in parallel bars against resistance to strengthen his gait pattern.

at the institute. I remained semi-conscious—comatose with failing BP vital signs for some time. The attending physicians informed my wife that I might not pull through the day.

She immediately telephoned my brother and sister.

In 16 hours I rallied and recovered.

If I live long enough, and if my physical condition permits, I shall write about the "how" of communication during this apparent terminal episode, of course based on my wife's observation and experience.